618.92 PRE c.2
Premature babies : a guide for parents /
CLAIBORNE PARISH LIBRARY
3 3838 00038 7500

PREMATURE BABIES

Y0-GEA-304

HAYNESVILLE
618.92
Premature babies.
c.2
15.95

DATE DUE			
MAY 18 '87			
JUL 22 '87			
JUL 1[illegible] 199[illegible]			
JUL 29 199[illegible]			
JUN 12 '92			
AU[illegible] 8 '9[illegible]			

CLAIBORNE PARISH LIBRARY
HOMER, LOUISIANA

Robert, who was tube-fed, is now a fine three year old in this family picture.

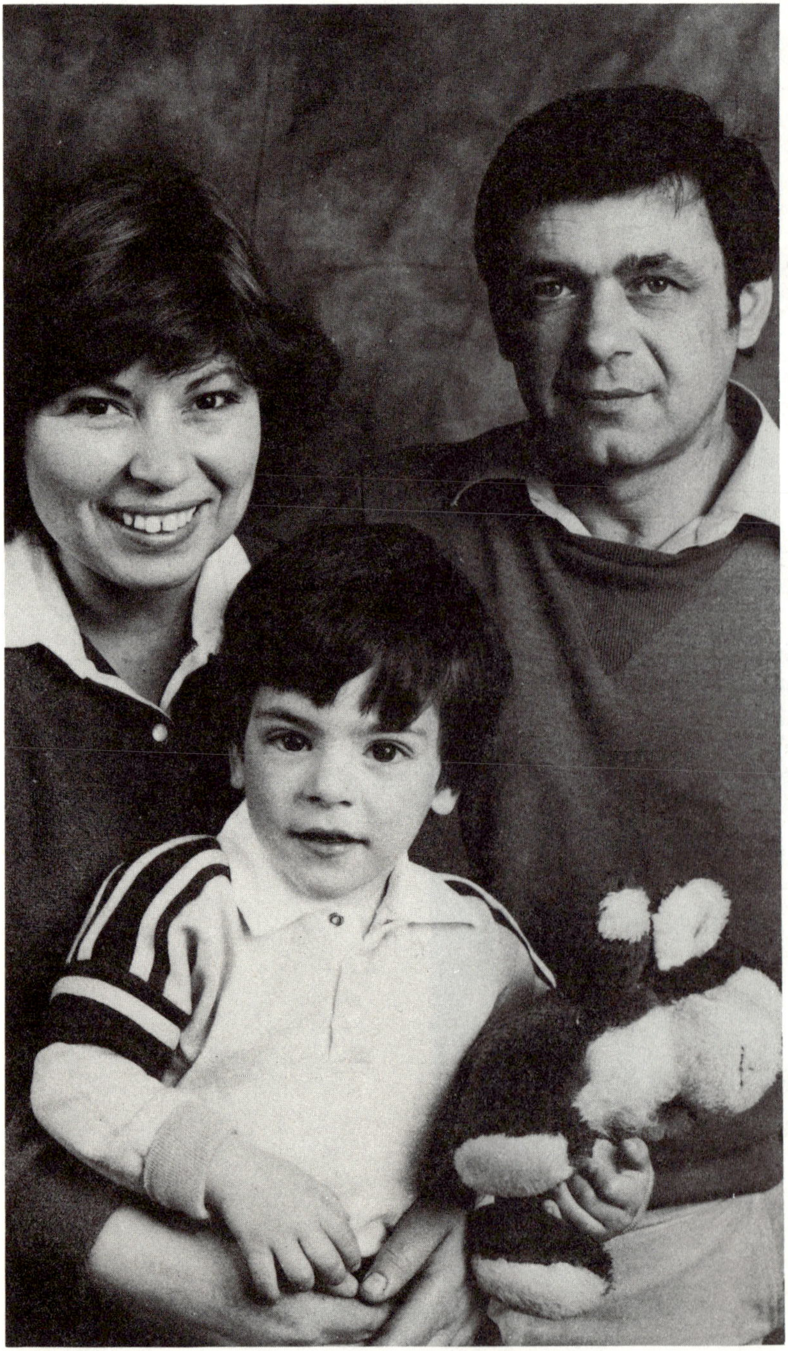

PREMATURE BABIES
A GUIDE FOR PARENTS

Dr W H Kitchen   M M Ryan   A L Rickards   J V Lissenden

Rodale Press, Emmaus, Pa.

Copyright © 1983 by W. H. Kitchen and M. M. Ryan

First published in Australia by Hill of Content
Publishing Company Pty Ltd

All rights reserved. No part of this publication may be reproduced or transmitted in any form or by any means, electronic or mechanical, including photocopy, recording, or any information storage and retrieval system, without the written permission of the publisher.

Printed in the United States of America on recycled paper containing a high percentage of de-inked fiber.

Cover art and design by Csaba Banki

Library of Congress Cataloging in Publication Data
Main entry under title:

Premature babies.

Bibliography: p.
1. Infants (Premature) 2. Infants (Premature) – Care and hygiene. I. Kitchen, W. H. (William Henry), 1926- . II. Title. [DNLM: 1. Infant, Premature – popular works. WS 420 P925]
RJ250.P72 1983 618.92'011 84-27675
ISBN 0-87857-557-X paperback

2 4 6 8 10 9 7 5 3 1 paperback

Contents

PREFACE

Why a book about premature babies?

Parents are increasingly interested in learning more about their babies, so parent education is now an accepted part of antenatal care. There are a number of excellent books available that explain to parents what they may expect of their baby immediately after birth and in the days, months and years that follow. However, most of this information concerns infants who are born close to the expected time.

Parents of premature infants have great difficulty in finding books that give the information **they** seek. Many of the publications on this subject are written by specialists for specialists and are difficult for parents to understand because of the numerous technical words used. They do not address the issues that are of immediate concern to the parents of a premature baby.

This book has been written to meet the need for more information. The authors have the varied professional backgrounds of nurse-midwife, social worker, psychologist and paediatrician, and in each case experience with their own children has added practical know-how to theoretical knowledge.

The most important people who have helped us with this book are the parents of premature babies. Over the years, fathers, mothers and other members of family have shared with us their fears and worries as well as their satisfactions and successes. They have given generously of their time and shown us many ways in which the care of such families might be improved. In a very real sense these people have asked the questions, given many of the answers and persuaded us that this information should be shared.

Although the doctors and nurses caring for a premature baby make a special effort to keep parents well informed about their baby's progress and problems, some parents still complain of great difficulty in either obtaining or understanding information. This book, then, is designed to give a general guide to parents — and immediate relatives — who are facing the crisis that surrounds the birth of a premature infant. However, a book has one great disadvantage for it 'talks to' rather than 'talks with' parents. So parents are asked to note that **this book is not a substitute for discussions of the details of your own baby with doctor and nurse. They will be expecting to answer your questions and will devote as much time as possible to this**

important part of your baby's welfare. This book provides you with background information and explanations that will help to make your conversations with the medical personnel easier and more meaningful.

Usually, friends and relatives, particularly the infant's grand-parents, offer great comfort and support to worried parents, but there are times when lack of knowledge and experience may make their advice either misleading or unhelpful. A chapter titled 'Family and Friends. How can they help?' is included especially and this may be shared with close friends and relatives as well as immediate members of the family.

Throughout the text, the personal pronoun 'he' is used almost exclusively for the premature baby, although the authors are well aware that about half of all babies are female. It was decided to adhere to this established grammatical convention, rather than to lengthen the text and make reading more difficult, by inserting 'he or she' on every occasion.

The authors wish to thank all the parents who have talked to us about their children, who suggested alterations and additions to the text and allowed us to publish their photographs. Dr Rose-mary C. Schwarz assisted in the preparation of Chapters 5 and 6 and the Teaching Aids Department of the Royal Women's Hospital, Melbourne, provided illustrations.

Dr W H Kitchen
Paediatrician

M M Ryan
Social Worker

A L Rickards
Clinical and Research Psychologist

J V Lissenden
Nurse-Midwife,

How to use this book

Parents reading this book for the first time soon after the birth of a premature baby may be so shocked and disturbed by their recent experience that the following important messages are all they will want to know for the moment:

- Most babies who weigh over a kilogram (almost $2\frac{1}{4}$ pounds) will live.
- Premature babies are small, but they are born at a time when the body is fully formed, even in such small details as finger and toe-nails.
- Parents of premature babies are usually very worried and anxious and this is normal. Nurses, doctors and others in the nursery find that many parents are very upset.
- Ask questions. If you don't understand, keep asking your questions; it is your right to know.
- Doctors and nurses will try to be honest with you. If there are special worries with your baby, you will be told.

Should parents read the whole book?

When you are ready, we suggest that you read only the sections that interest you and apply to your baby. Many parents will not need to read the book from cover to cover.

Each chapter has the most important information at the beginning. Read the remainder — for more information — when you are ready. You may wish to leave the more detailed sections until another time.

The doctors and nurses looking after your baby will explain about equipment used to help your baby and the difficulties that premature babies may have after birth. You may find it helps to read about these matters in the book and you may like to make a list of questions to ask the doctor or nurse later.

Parents' needs differ in regard to information. Some are happy to have only a general understanding of what is happening and don't wish to know any details or have technical explanations. If this is how **you** feel, it is fine. Other parents may like to know as much as possible. Your needs will be met by talking with the nursery staff and by reading the parts of this book that concern you; later perhaps, you may wish to look at some of the other published material mentioned at the end of the book.

Very often one parent (usually the mother) will have more opportunities than the other parent to talk with the medical and nursing staff about their baby. However they may find it difficult to pass on the information gained to their partner. Appropriate sections of this book may be most helpful in this regard.

CHAPTER 1 Why is our baby small?

Most newborn babies weigh about 3500 grams, or 7½ pounds. Usually birth takes place about 40 weeks (9 months) from the first day of the last menstrual period. This is often called 'term' or 'the expected date of delivery'. About one baby in every twenty weighs less than 2500 grams (5½ pounds) and most of these infants are cared for in a 'premature' or 'special care' nursery.

All small babies are not the same. The 'true premature' infant is born early and is small just because there has not been enough time for growth to take place. For example, after 28 weeks from the last period, the average baby has grown to 1000 grams (2¼ pounds) and by 36 weeks, the average weight is only 2500 grams (5½ pounds).

Some babies are born close to the expected time but are very small because growth in the womb has been very slow indeed. These poorly grown babies are usually called 'small-for-dates'. Intrauterine growth retardation, dysmature or placental insufficiency are alternative words for the same condition.

It is important to make this separation into true premature infants and small-for-dates infants because they behave differently in some important ways. An example will help to make this clearer. Some completely normal, healthy adults are no larger than an average 14 year old child yet the two are obviously completely different despite their similarity in size.

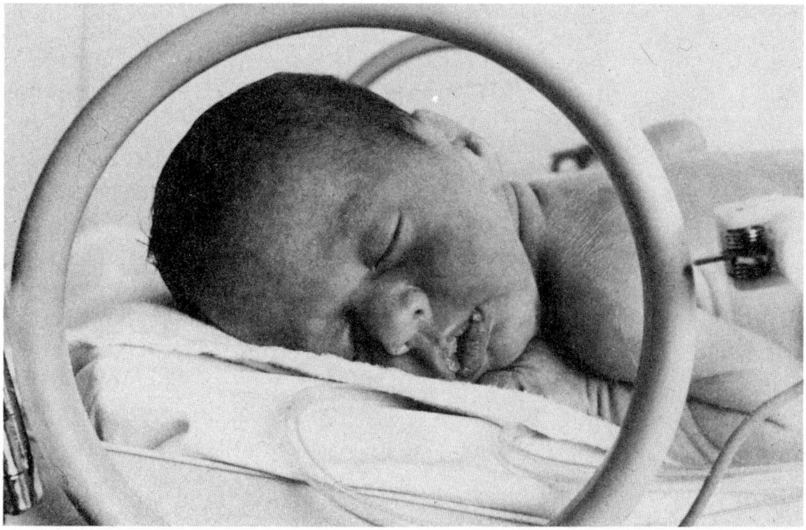

George, viewed through the porthole of his incubator, weighed 1760 grams at birth and was 7 weeks premature. He has sucking blisters on his lips, a common occurrence in young babies.

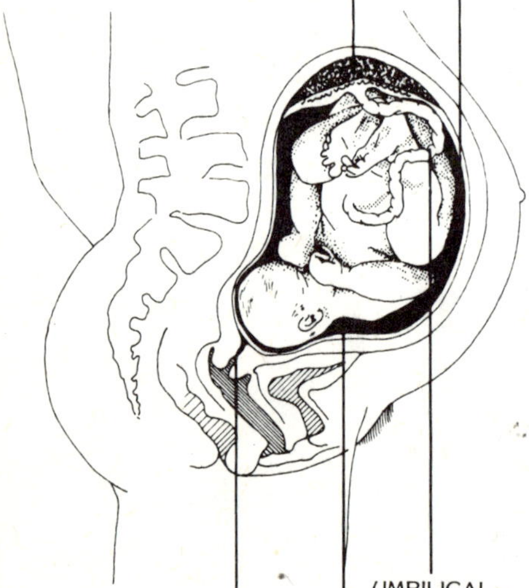

The unborn baby in the uterus

Gestation and gestational age

Doctors and nurses often use the term 'gestation' to indicate the number of weeks that the baby has developed in the uterus (womb) before birth. A 9 month or 'term baby' has a gestational age of 40 weeks; a baby who is born 3 months prematurely has a gestation (gestational age) of 28 weeks.

Why did my baby come early?

Most parents ask themselves why they had a premature baby and wonder whether either of them is to blame in any way. Premature labour is seldom anybody's fault and particularly not that of the parents.

What causes premature labour?

Often the cause for premature labour is unknown; sometimes there is a definite medical reason:

(a) **Twins and triplets** are very often born early.

(b) **'The waters' may break early** (premature rupture of the membranes). Normally the sac of fluid (liquor) surrounding the developing baby does not break until shortly before the baby is born when labour starts at about the expected date (term). Sometimes, the 'waters' break many weeks earlier than the expected time and the mother usually comes into labour hours or days later.

(c) **Neck of womb opens** (cervical incompetence)
Normally the neck of the womb (cervix) remains tightly closed until labour starts at term. Sometimes the neck of the womb begins to open up many weeks before the due date. The 'waters' may break and labour start. This is an important cause of premature delivery that can often be prevented next pregnancy by a 'cervical stitch'. In suitable cases, the obstetrician ties a piece of thread around the neck of the womb, quite early in the pregnancy; this helps that pregnancy to go to term.

(d) **Bleeding of the 'after-birth'** (placenta) Sometimes the

premature labour is caused by a small amount of bleeding which separates the after-birth from the wall of the womb.
This is called an 'accidental haemorrhage' and, as the name implies, cannot be prevented and is nobody's fault.

(e) **Baby brought on early** (deliberate action because of some illness in the mother that makes it unwise for the pregnancy to continue.) Occasionally, labour is brought on (induced) because the unborn baby is becoming increasingly sick, for example in the case of severe Rh disease, or when special tests show the baby is not growing and it is therefore safer for him to be born, even if premature.

(f) **Abnormalities of the womb are occasionally the cause of premature labour.** Your obstetrician would know about any such abnormality and should explain it to you in detail.

It should be repeated that sometimes no cause for premature labour can be found. In this situation many mothers continue to worry that something they or their partner has done has caused the premature birth. If you have any special worry of this kind, no matter how illogical it may seem, ask about it. There are many 'old wives tales' that have caused some mothers of premature babies a great deal of unnecessary worry.

Why is a baby small-for-dates?

(a) The baby may be very small but born close to the expected date if the mother has high blood pressure (essential hyper-tension) or 'kidney-trouble' (pre-eclampsia) during pregnancy. Normally the mother would be well aware that she had these conditions.

(b) Small mothers fortunately often have small babies; usually they are taller than their mother when they grow up.

(c) Occasionally a baby is small-for-dates because of a virus infection that started long before birth, such as German measles (rubella).

(d) Sometimes small-for-dates babies have a serious malformation. This is usually very obvious as soon as the baby is born and your doctor will have discussed this with you.

(e) Heavy cigarette smoking, excessive alcohol during pregnancy and narcotic addiction sometimes result in a small baby.

(f) Sometimes the placenta (after-birth) is not transferring enough 'food' from mother to developing baby to allow normal growth to continue.

Sometimes there is a combination of several of these conditions. As you read these lists of causes, it is obvious that the birth of a very small infant is seldom the parents' fault. If you are worried that smoking, alcohol or drugs were to blame, this should be discussed with your doctor.

Parents' thoughts on the reasons for premature birth

In the days and weeks after the baby's birth, many parents spend much time trying to think of the cause. It seems to be in our nature to try to find a cause. Some parents place the blame on doctor or nurse-midwife, usually unjustly; many mothers blame themselves, almost always incorrectly. To the outsider the 'cause' they settle on may seem trivial and illogical, for example, failure to take medicine as prescribed or eating unusual food. On other occasions, the father may be blamed, again, often unjustly.

The question of 'cause of prematurity' is one that you must discuss with your doctor or nurse so that, as parents, you are not assuming blame that is unjust and illogical. Some parents are embarrassed to mention their ideas about possible causes of premature labour because they fear that they will appear foolish. Medical and nursing attendants expect to be asked these questions; they will take them seriously and will give you an answer if it is known. However, there are some controversial areas; these include the influence, if any, of sexual intercourse during pregnancy and of a previous termination of pregnancy. If you are concerned, we can only repeat our earlier advice to discuss the matter with your doctor.

CHAPTER 2 Will my baby live?

This is likely to be your first and most important question and only time will answer it for you. Your paediatrician is the one to give you information on your baby's chances.

The majority of babies entering a neonatal intensive care unit eventually go home. In recent years, the care of very small infants has made tremendous advances. Admittedly, very few babies who are more than 14 weeks premature survive, but at each week after that the chances improve with increasing gestational age. Most babies who are less than eight weeks premature will live.

The weight and degree of prematurity of your baby are not the only factors used by the doctor to assess chances of survival. Some infants have severe difficulty with breathing, or are suffering from the effects of oxygen lack during labour or have a serious malformation. Your doctor will know if your baby has any of these conditions. On the other hand, some infants are unusually free of trouble and there is room for greater optimism.

When will the 'danger' or critical period be over?

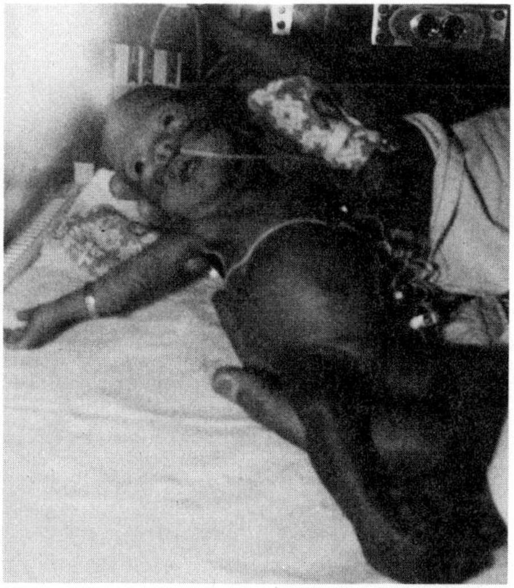

This is Carlie who weighed 860 grams at birth. She is shown here in her father's hands with his wedding ring around her wrist.

Parents often ask this question and the paediatrician may find it a hard one to answer. The first day of life is by far the most dangerous time and most of the deaths occur before two weeks. If your infant reaches this age you would be most unfortunate not to take him home eventually. There is an important exception. Infants needing ventilator support are not really 'out of the woods' until they are breathing entirely without help and the lungs have returned to normal. Even so, about 70 per cent of infants who are sick enough to need ventilator treatment recover fully.

Do not hesitate to ask your doctor for his estimate of the baby's chance of living. A few doctors will not mention this unless you ask. It is also important to remember that the first day is the most dangerous time, and thereafter the outlook usually gets steadily better. Admittedly, unexpected complications may sometimes turn up later, but you and your doctor will then talk about their importance.

CHAPTER 3 Difficulties premature babies may have

This chapter gives more technical information on the difficulties mentioned in the previous chapter. It is suggested that you read the sections that apply to your own baby rather than read about all the problems, most of which you may not meet at all.

Early development

When a baby is born prematurely, basic functions such as sucking, swallowing, and digestion of milk are poorly developed. A baby who is born early does not speed up his development; on the contrary he matures at about the same rate as in the uterus and he will not behave like a term baby until he reaches the expected time of birth. For example, a baby who is born ten weeks early (at thirty weeks) usually will not learn to suck vigorously and behave like a healthy newborn infant until he is eight to ten weeks old.

Feeding behaviour

If your baby was born three or four weeks early, usually there will be only minor difficulties. He could be a little sleepy and not very interested in taking the breast or bottle; or you may find his sucking less vigorous. With extra help from nursing staff and persistence and understanding on the mother's part, these temporary minor troubles should be overcome so that full breast or bottle feeding is possible; usually, your baby spends just a little extra time in hospital. With this slight degree of prematurity, you may want to get some help at home from a nurse, family member, or an infant care helper if you are not fully confident when ready to leave the hospital.

If the baby is more than four weeks premature, greater temporary difficulties may be expected. Infants between four and eight weeks early usually manage to suck some of their feeds from a bottle in the first two or three days of life. At this stage, the baby only requires small amounts of food. Gradually, as his feeds are increased in line with his bodily needs, he will tire and be unable to take his full quota. The baby who is too tired to suck is 'tube-fed'. This is also called 'gavage feeding'. You will be able to watch this type of feeding in the nursery. Tube feeding is performed by a specially trained nurse who gently passes a fine plastic tube through the baby's mouth into his stomach. Then a funnel or syringe is connected to this plastic tube and the milk slowly runs into the infant's stomach. The feeding (gavage) tube is then gently removed. Tube feeding does not upset the baby or damage the gullet; it makes sure that the baby gets enough milk to thrive. When the mother of a tube fed baby feels comfortable with the idea, she may like to help with the tube feeding.

Tube feeding does not teach or encourage a baby to be 'lazy'. About two weeks before the 'expected date of birth', most infants begin 'to fight gavage'. They are restless, suck on the tube and toss their heads around during the tube feed. This is the signal for which the nurse has been waiting. For a few days, the nurse gives the first part of the feed by gavage and then encourages the baby to suck the remainder from a bottle. Sometimes 'alternate gavage and bottle' is given, allowing the baby to suck one feed and then to be tube fed next time. As soon as a baby begins to suck from the bottle the mother usually will be able to help with some bottle feeds.

If the baby is more than four weeks premature he is unlikely to do well at the breast and will be best managed by skilled nurses with tube feeding. Sometimes babies who are not ready to suckle are put to the breast to help mother and baby get to know each other. The infant often does not suck, or only poorly, but gradually breast feeds will improve. This practice of having baby at mother's breast is often called 'skin contact'. Both mother and baby enjoy the skin contact even if little or no milk is taken.

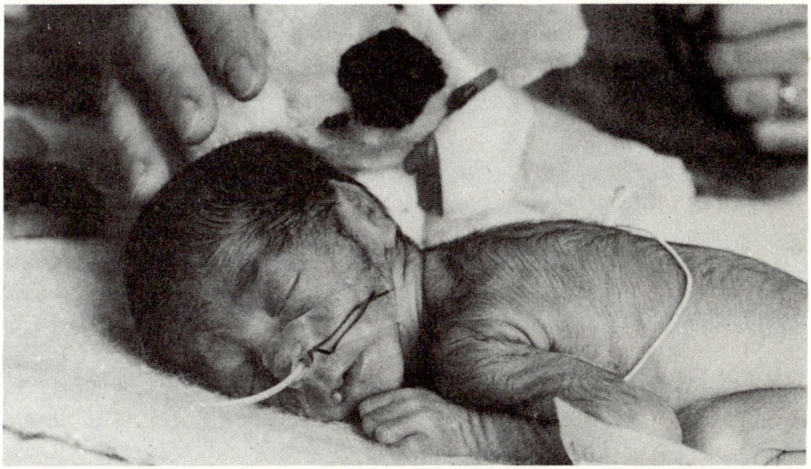

Joseph weighs 1020 grams, he is 2 weeks old in the picture and has a fine covering of hair (lanugo), normal for premature babies. He is not able to suck yet so the tube in his nose goes to his stomach. He needs some milk every hour.

Infants more than eight weeks premature can be expected to have more troubles with feeding in the first few weeks than those less premature, but again, fortunately there are many ways to overcome these difficulties. The very small baby sucks so weakly that bottle or breast feeding is quite impossible. These very small babies may not even be able to swallow. Also the capacity of the stomach is so small that a big feed cannot be given or the baby will vomit. Finally, the rest of the bowel has not yet developed good powers of propelling the food or of normal digestion, so these babies readily vomit, or the stomach (abdomen) becomes rather large (distended), unless feedings are very small and frequent.

Sometimes the plastic gavage tube is left in position so that feeding can be given every two hours, or every hour, or even as a continuous trickle of milk all the time. If the tube is left down all the time, it will be lightly strapped to the baby's face. Sometimes it is put through the nose, not the mouth. This is because it is harder for the baby to accidentally pull out the feeding tube from his nose.

Some babies are not able to take sufficient milk to meet their growth needs and a few are not able to feed at all. It is now common to give some, or even all the food requirements of these babies, into a vein — a method called 'intravenous alimentation'. These babies are then able to grow until they are large and mature enough to be fed by mouth. Intravenous feeding is a very complicated technique and it requires highly skilled nurses, doctors and a good laboratory if it is to be used safely. It is only used if simpler methods of feeding are inadequate, or the baby is very premature.

What milk is given to the baby?

Premature babies may be successfully reared on a variety of milk feedings. Human breast milk has a lot of advantages and if ample supplies are available, many doctors favour the use of breast milk (see Chapter 4). If your expressed breast milk can be delivered fresh and scrupulously clean to the nursery, usually it is possible to give your milk to your own baby. Also breast milk can be deep-frozen and kept until your baby needs it. Some nurseries collect breast milk from all mothers in one container, sterilize it and then use this for all babies. This is called 'pooled breast milk'. If adequate supplies of breast milk are not available, it is usual that some or all of the feed will be of cow's milk origin and babies make good progress on this. If the mother is not attempting to breast feed, a satisfactory artificial substitute will be found.

Jaundice

More than half of all babies develop jaundice (a yellow colour of the skin). If your baby is jaundiced you will notice that he has a yellow colour of the skin, almost reminding you of a suntan. It should be emphasized that many jaundiced babies need no treatment at all because the jaundice is so mild. For those who develop deep jaundice, effective treatment is readily available.

All newborn babies have more red blood cells than they need after birth; this unwanted blood is broken down into a yellow-coloured chemical called 'bilirubin' and this colours the skin, eyes and urine yellow. This yellow-coloured bilirubin is removed from the blood by the liver. In the first few days of life, the process is not very efficient for this is a job that the liver did not have to do before the baby's birth. It takes a few days for the liver to work really well in a normal sized baby; in the premature baby even more time is required for the liver to work efficiently and to clear the jaundice. Some mothers are needlessly worried that their baby may 'catch' jaundice in the nursery. It is **not** infectious.

Jaundice in premature babies **is not dangerous** if it is carefully managed. This the doctor and nurse will certainly do. The depth of yellow colour of the baby is not a very good guide to the importance of jaundice. If your doctor is at all concerned about the jaundice, he will arrange to do a blood test (serum bilirubin) once or twice a day until it is definitely getting better.

Phototherapy

If the jaundice in a baby is moderate, the paediatrician may use treatment with fluorescent lights to clear it more quickly. This is called phototherapy and is often used in special care nurseries. The yellow substance (bilirubin) in the baby's blood is broken down if the skin is exposed to bright light from several fluorescent light tubes.

Anna is having phototherapy, above her are the fluorescent tubes; she lies naked except for protective covers over her eyes. Anna was only 4 weeks premature but weighed 3500 g because her mother is a diabetic.

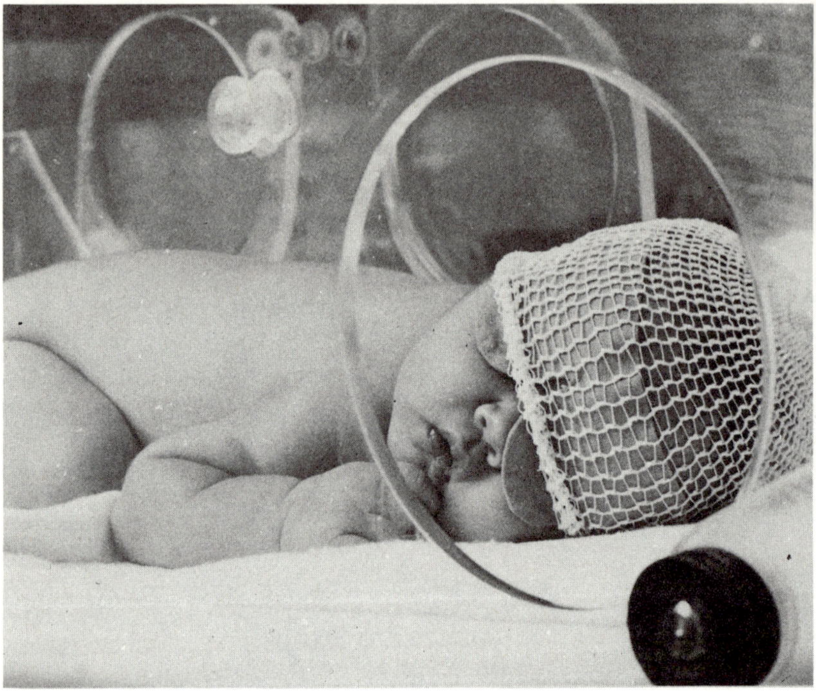

The photograph shows a baby having phototherapy. So that light can reach as much of the skin as possible, she is naked – not even a diaper. The skin on front and back of the body is exposed to the lights by frequent turning of the baby. You will note that the eyes are covered to protect them from bright light; however, these eye covers occasionally slip off and this brief exposure to light does not matter. Babies under phototherapy or 'light treatment' often get loose green bowel actions because the substance formed by the breakdown of the bilirubin is green in colour and it finishes up in the bowel. The green colour shows that the light treatment is working. Many larger babies having phototherapy develop a fine rash because they are sweating under the lights. This rash soon goes once treatment ceases. As these babies are sweating, they need extra water so extra feedings may be given.

If the jaundice is due to prematurity only, phototherapy is often the only treatment needed. At other times jaundice may be made worse because of bruising or because the mother and baby have a different blood group (blood group incompatibility). Your paediatrician would know of these or any unusual causes of jaundice.

Exchange transfusion

Occasionally phototherapy alone will not control the jaundice so another type of treatment is used. This is called an exchange transfusion and it may need to be performed more than once. Your paediatrician would explain the need for an exchange transfusion and talk about the small risk that goes with it. An exchange transfusion is usually performed by putting a small plastic tube into the big vein in the baby's umbilicus (navel). The doctor then draws out about 10 ml (about $\frac{1}{3}$ ounce) of blood, discards it, and then injects exactly the same amount of fresh blood obtained from the blood bank. This withdrawal and replacement of blood is repeated many times. The blood withdrawn from the baby contains a lot of bilirubin (the cause of the jaundice) whereas the blood from the blood-bank is free of all jaundice. This replacement of jaundiced baby's blood by donor blood helps greatly to reduce this condition. The blood used for the exchange transfusion comes from adult donors to the blood bank; your baby's blood group is always checked and the laboratory makes certain that the donor blood is suitable for your baby.

Some parents are worried that the baby will be changed in some way because of this transfusion, but there is no need for concern. The donor blood gradually wears out over the next three months and it is entirely replaced by new blood that the baby has made in the normal way. There is no permanent change at all.

Earlier it was stated that jaundice was not dangerous if carefully managed and you will now realize that there is effective treatment available. If jaundice is allowed to become very deep and remains untreated serious troubles occasionally may arise. Before phototherapy and exchange transfusions were available, deep jaundice sometimes resulted in cerebral palsy ('spasticity') or deafness. This is the reason that jaundice is now treated.

Keeping warm

The premature baby can become cold very easily, partly because he is so small. He also has very little fat under his skin. (Fat is a good insulator; it keeps seals and whales warm in icy water.) The nursing staff will spend a lot of time maintaining the body warmth of your premature baby. The smaller the infant, the more care is needed. The methods used are:

(a) **Warm cot.** If the baby is only three or four weeks premature, hot water bottles or an electric blanket are used in an ordinary cot to keep the baby warm. It is important that the room is warm too, so a specially heated nursery is essential. The nurse will take the baby's temperature frequently and supply more or less heat as necessary. The baby is changed as quickly as possible and not unwrapped more often than is absolutely essential.

(b) **Closed incubator.** Infants who are very premature or will not keep warm in an ordinary cot are placed in a plastic-walled incubator. Inside the incubator, the air is very warm and a fan keeps it circulating. Again the baby's temperature is taken regularly and the nurse adjusts the incubator control to make the air in the incubator a little warmer or cooler to suit individual needs. One form of this incubator has a little pad taped on to the baby and the temperature of the incubator is automatically adjusted by the baby's skin temperature — this system is called 'servo-control'.

Babies in incubators are often left naked except for a diaper. In this way they can be observed easily and breathing is not hindered at all. You may find that a sheet of bubble plastic or a semicircular sheet of plastic has been placed over the baby. This acts like a blanket and helps the baby to keep warm, but still allows the staff to see that colour and breathing are satisfactory.

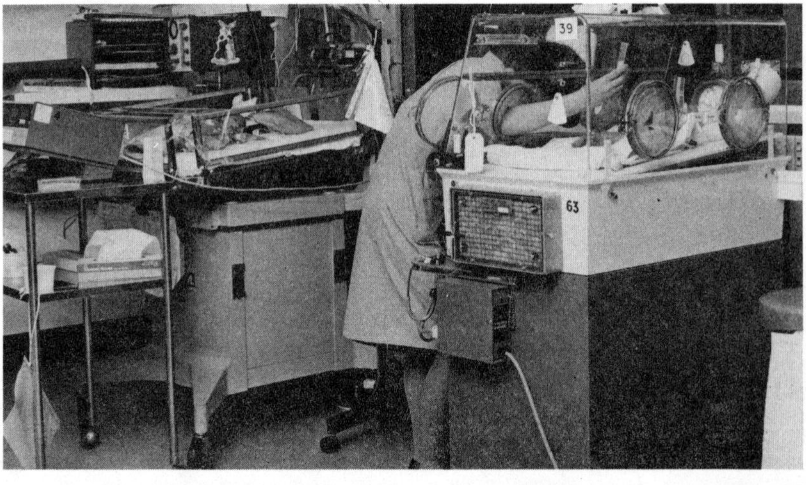

This is an incubator of the closed type. Michelle is being tube-fed by one of the nursery sisters.

(c) **Open incubators.** These are used for very small or very sick babies. As there are no doors or 'portholes' to open, it is much easier for the nurses to look after those babies who need constant attention. The baby lies naked on a mattress and above is a heating element which beams heat down onto the baby. There is a small thermometer taped to the baby's body which automatically tells the electric heater just how much heat output is needed.

Although this is the most recent type of incubator available, it is not necessary for every premature baby to be nursed in this way. In fact, many infants do better in a closed incubator and are therefore nursed there.

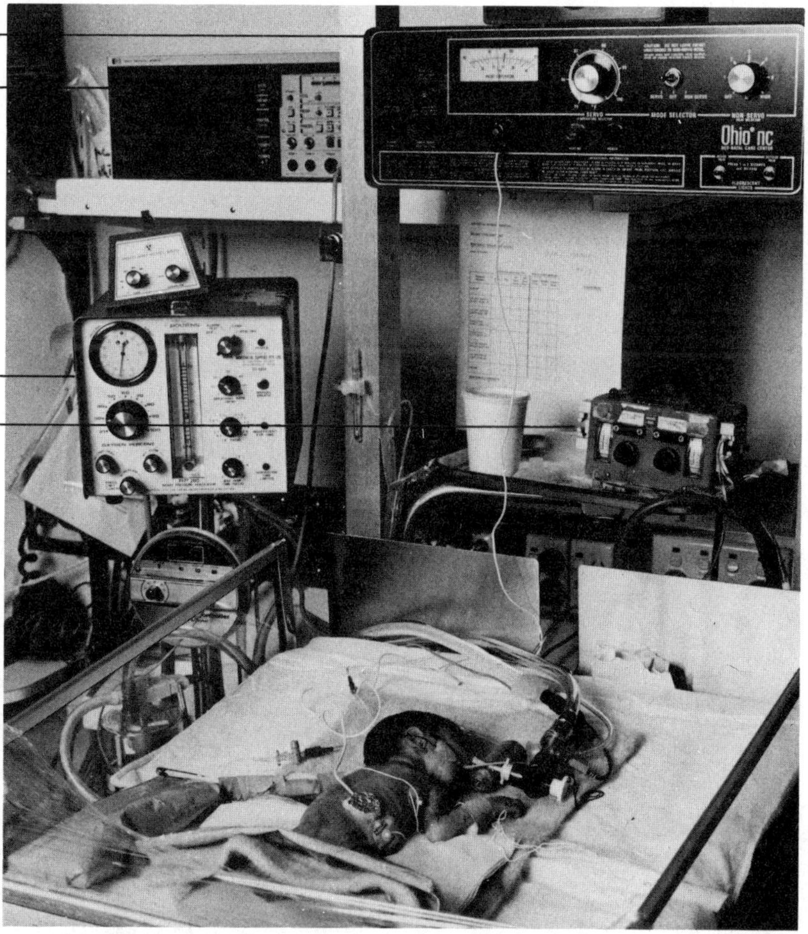

Peter weighs 920 grams (about 2 lbs) and is in an open incubator. He was born 13 weeks prematurely.

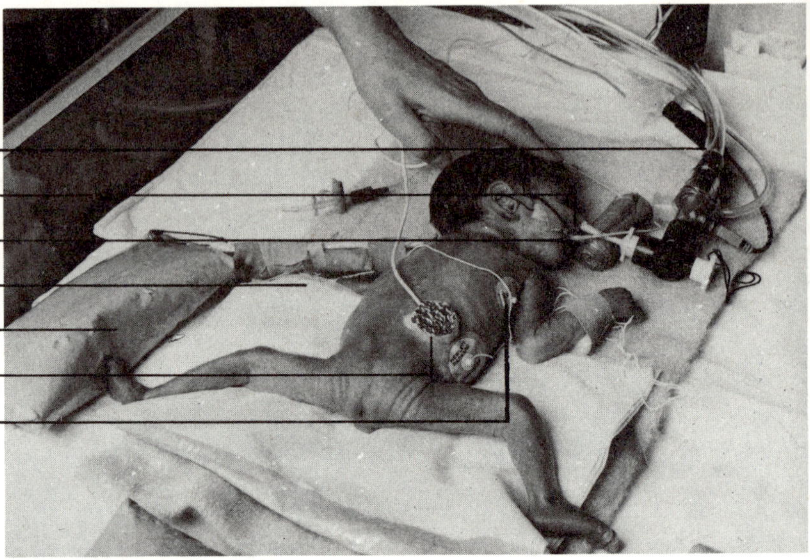

Breathing difficulties (Respiratory Distress)

The lungs of a baby born at term (nine months or forty weeks) are well developed, they expand at birth and air is able to be breathed efficiently.

The premature baby has lungs that are only partly developed and some trouble with breathing is very common. Again, there is a great deal that can be done to assist the premature baby with breathing troubles.

Premature babies with breathing problems breathe quickly. They often make a grunting noise on breathing out; the ribs and lower part of the breast-bone are sucked in as the baby breathes in. These babies may need more oxygen than is present in the air we breathe to remain a pink, healthy colour. This difficulty with breathing is called Respiratory Distress Syndrome or R.D.S. for short. Often the breathing problem lasts only a few hours and your paediatrician will call it 'wet lung' or 'transient tachypnoea'.

Sometimes it lasts longer and then it is usually called 'hyaline membrane disease' or 'idiopathic respiratory distress'. These names are mentioned because many doctors and nurses use them in speaking to parents so it will be helpful to know what they mean.

Wet lung (transient tachypnoea) means that the lungs, filled with fluid until birth, have been a little slow in getting rid of the excess water. However this clears satisfactorily after a few hours and breathing settles to the normal rate of about forty breaths per minute.

Hyaline Membrane Disease is a more serious condition, but again there is effective treatment available. If your baby has hyaline membrane disease, it is worthwhile understanding more about it. Healthy lungs are rather like a bunch of grapes except that the grapes and all the stalks are hollow and filled with air. The 'skin' of each individual 'grape', called alveolus, is covered with blood capillaries that pick up oxygen and get rid of carbon dioxide. In the infant with hyaline membrane disease the individual grapes collapse when the baby breathes out instead of staying partly open as in our bunch of grapes analogy. This means that every time the baby breathes in, he has to expand his lungs completely from an almost airless state. This makes breathing very hard work. In mild cases of hyaline membrane disease it takes two or three days for the lungs to return to a normal state where the alveoli stay open when the infant breathes out.

In the meantime, the following help may be given:

(a) **Extra oxygen** is put into the incubator or a head box enclosing the baby's head. The air we breathe contains about 21 per cent of oxygen, oxygen being essential to life. Babies with mild hyaline membrane disease, often need to breathe air with the oxygen concentration increased to 30 per cent or 40 per cent whilst infants with severe breathing difficulties may even require 'pure oxygen' (concentration of 100 per cent).

(b) **Feeding is needed** because the baby is working very hard, using a lot of energy for breathing. Sometimes 'tube' or bottle feeding is possible, but many babies have a few days on a simple type of intravenous feeding with water and glucose.

(c) **Testing of blood**. To make sure that the amount of oxygen in the blood is not too high or too low, small amounts of blood are tested frequently. Sometimes the sample of blood is obtained from a plastic tube passed into an artery of the baby's navel (umbilicus) and called an 'umbilical artery catheter'. Blood may

The head box inside the incubator makes sure that Paul gets the extra oxygen he needs. Paul was 12 weeks premature and has already doubled his birthweight.

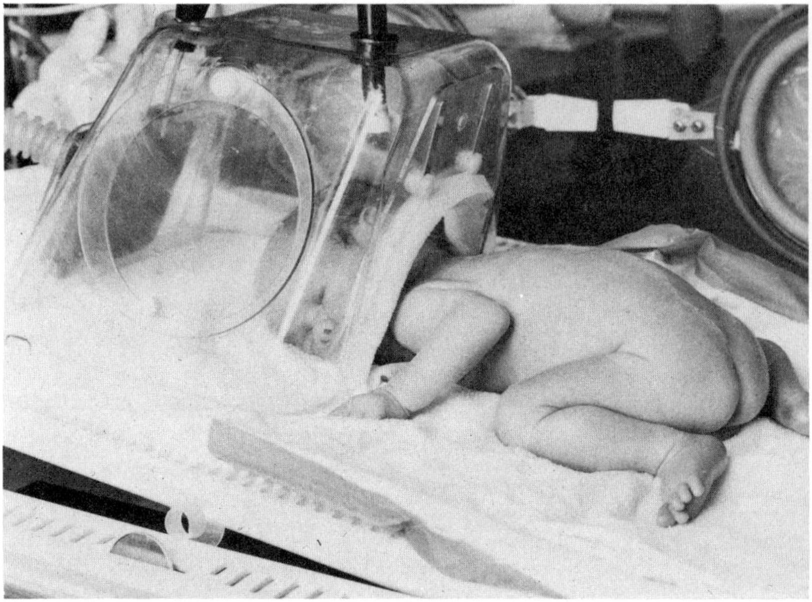

also be obtained from an artery at the wrist (radial artery). Oxygen in the blood can also be measured by means of a small instrument placed on the baby's skin. This is called a trans-cutaneous oxygen monitor. This 'skin sensor' is heated to increase the blood supply to the skin so that a temporary red spot remains on the skin when the sensor is removed.

(d) **CPAP**. If the hyaline membrane disease is moderately severe, the baby may be given a very helpful treatment called continuous positive airway pressure or CPAP. The principle is simple. You will remember that in hyaline membrane disease the lungs collapse when the baby breathes out. If a small pressure is kept in the lungs all the time, the lung collapse is prevented and the baby has a much easier time breathing. There are several ways of applying this pressure, so, if your baby is having CPAP, ask the doctor or nurse to explain how it is being given.

(e) **Ventilator treatment.** Many babies with hyaline membrane disease begin to improve after two or three days.

However a few infants get steadily worse and it is necessary for a machine, called a ventilator, to take over the baby's breathing. Usually a plastic tube is passed through the nose down into the windpipe (trachea) and this is connected to the ventilator.

This type of treatment is needed for the more severe cases. About one in every four of all babies who need ventilation develop a pneumothorax when air leaks out of the lungs. A chest drain is then required. An infant on a ventilator certainly may have a long and difficult time before he is able to breathe again by himself and it must be admitted that a few do not survive. Your doctor will explain about your individual baby's chances.

Once a baby is on a ventilator, some complications are almost certain to occur and parents would be told about them and their importance.

Apnoea (The word means 'not breathing')

In the very small infant there may be times when breathing becomes shallow or temporarily stops, the heart beat becomes slower and the skin colour turns slightly blue. The simple explanation is that the very immature baby just 'forgets' to breathe. As there are sometimes other causes, it is usual to do some special tests on these infants.

These 'dusky turns', or 'apnoeic attacks', are common in very small babies and the experienced nurse is highly skilled in their management. Usually, to make breathing start again, it is merely necessary to give the baby a gentle shake or move him a little, or stimulate the skin (cutaneous stimulation).

In a special care nursery, electronic equipment is available to watch over the baby's breathing rather than relying entirely on the nurses' continuous observation. The 'apnoea alarm' is a simple machine which is not attached to the baby. The baby lies on a special mattress or pad and an electronic device sounds an alarm if the mattress ceases to move in the event of breathing becoming very shallow or ceasing.

A 'cardio-respiratory monitor' is sometimes used to continuously check that the baby's heart rate and breathing are normal. This type of monitor is connected to the skin of the baby's chest by three thin wires attached to small metal discs. If breathing or heart slows, an alarm sounds or flashes and the baby receives immediate attention from the nurse.

Treatment of mild apnoeic attacks only requires the baby to be disturbed or 'stimulated' so that breathing starts again. If these mild attacks are happening very frequently, a medicine called theophylline (elixophylline) may be given. Often, very small babies with frequent or severe apnoeic attacks are managed by using a ventilator for a few days.

Infection

Premature babies sometimes pick up infections in the womb before birth if the waters broke many hours before delivery. Occasionally, the premature baby will pick up an infection after birth and this may occur no matter how scrupulously careful the staff and parents are with cleanliness and care of the baby.

The medical staff are always very careful to detect and to treat infection in a premature baby. If antibiotics are given early, the trouble is usually cured. Often there are false alarms; infection may be suspected and antibiotics started, but later when the results of tests come back, no infection is found. Experience has shown that it is much safer to be very careful when there is the slightest suspicion of infection rather than to adopt a wait and see policy.

If your doctor suspects an infection, he will send several specimens to the laboratory for culture and if the result is reported as 'negative', there is no infection. If bacteria are grown, the laboratory performs 'sensitivity tests' which tell the doctor the most effective antibiotics to be used. Sometimes the final results of tests for infection are not available for a few days. Sometimes your baby will be moved to an isolation nursery to prevent the infection spreading to other babies.

Bleeding troubles

Premature babes seldom have difficulties because of bleeding. A few are rather bruised, even after a normal, careful delivery. This type of bruising may make the jaundice a little worse, but bruising and jaundice soon go.

Intraventricular Haemorrhage

In all humans the brain has central cavities (ventricles) that are normally filled with a clear watery fluid (cerebro-spinal fluid or C.S.F.).

Small babies, particularly those who weigh less than 1500 grams ($3\frac{3}{4}$ pounds) at birth may bleed into these cavities (ventricles) in the centre of the brain. This is called intraventricular haemorrhage. Understandably, parents are likely to be shocked and alarmed if they are told that their baby has a 'haemorrhage in the brain'. We would emphasize that this occurs frequently in small premature babies and very often the amount of bleeding is small and is not a real worry. Occasionally the bleeding is more serious. Your paediatrician will discuss this matter with you in detail.

Intraventricular haemorrhage is found by using a sonar machine — similar to the one used on many mothers to examine the unborn baby during pregnancy. This examination uses high frequency sound waves and does not harm the baby in any way. Sometimes a special type of x-ray machine called a 'CAT scan' is used instead of or in addition to the sonar examination.

If a baby has an intraventricular haemorrhage, it is usual to repeat the sonar examination to make sure that the central cavities of the brain are not becoming too big. If your baby has any haemorrhage or enlargement of the central cavities of the brain, your paediatrician would discuss this in detail with you.

Necrotizing enterocolitis

This is an inflammation of the bowel wall; the cause of this condition is uncertain. It is not a common complication. Mostly it happens in the very premature baby. Necrotizing enterocolitis (N.E.C.) is suspected if the baby gets a very distended abdomen (stomach) and sometimes there is blood in the bowel actions. Again, this is a problem that is often suspected and the baby may be x-rayed and feedings stopped for a time. Quite often this worry proves unnecessary, but it is better to be very careful rather than wait and see. Many infants with necrotizing enterocolitis get better after a few days of antibiotics and intravenous feeding but a few require an operation.

Patent ductus

This is a condition that often occurs in small babies with hyaline membrane disease. The 'ductus' is a large artery that has an important use to the unborn baby because it allows most of the blood to circulate without going through the lungs which obviously are not used for breathing air before birth. At the time of birth, as soon as the baby's lungs fill with air, the ductus normally closes so that immediately after birth the lungs have a good circulation of blood.

In small premature babies with hyaline membrane disease, the ductus may open up again for a time. Usually it closes itself later without treatment; sometimes a medication is given, or occasion ally the ductus has to be 'tied off' by the surgeon. If your baby has a patent ductus, your paediatrician will be able to explain if any treatment is planned.

Hernias

Many premature babies develop a hernia in the navel (umbilical hernia). Usually they need no treatment but occasionally there are some babies who may ultimately need an operation.

Some premature infants develop a hernia in one or both groins (inguinal hernia). These are more likely to need a surgical operation, but the results are excellent; babies tolerate these operations very well indeed. If you are concerned about the operation, make sure you have your questions answered.

A hernia is a weakness in the wall of the abdomen and through this hole some of the contents may come out under the skin. These hernias may look unsightly but usually are not painful to the baby. They are not a serious problem if medical advice is followed.

Difficulties with feeding, temperature maintenance, breathing, jaundice and apnoea are the most important problems facing the premature baby but you now realize that modern care has a great deal to offer for each of these troubles.

CHAPTER 4 Breast feeding

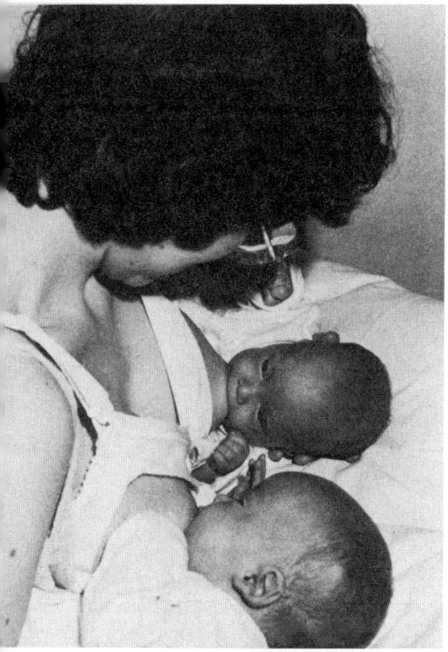

Roderick and Anthony are twins, they are 4 months old here and feeding at the breast together at last. Roderick weighed 1280 grams at birth and Anthony only 900 grams, so they were parted for quite a while.

Should you try to breast feed? Medical opinion suggests that breast milk, even for a short time, is helpful to your baby. Breast milk is most suitable for a baby because it contains all the nutrients in the correct amounts and is individually made by you for your baby. Breast milk also contains antibodies, white blood cells and other substances that protect against infection; these anti-infective properties are present in largest amounts in the 'colostrum'. This yellow fluid or 'first milk' is produced in only small amounts for the first three or four days after the birth of your baby, but it is especially important because of its protective qualities.

After the third day, the mother will know that the 'milk has come in' because her breasts are full and increasing amounts of milk are produced. This milk is high in protein and is particularly good for the premature baby for it is easily digested and also has important anti-infective properties. Both colostrum and breast milk retain many of their advantages even if stored by deep freezing.

More detailed information on the advantages of breast feeding can be found in books named at the end of this chapter.

Do not be discouraged as you read this chapter because it tells of the problems that may occur if you decide to breast feed your premature baby. Many mothers fully breast feed for as long as they wish and those who are not quite so successful usually can supply enough milk for a few weeks at least. Most of the difficulties are temporary and can be overcome with help and patience.

In Chapter 3, the difficulties a premature baby has in sucking and swallowing were described. By the time your baby has reached thirty-six to thirty-seven weeks of development you can expect him to suck at the breast, but not very well. By thirty-eight to thirty-nine weeks, many babies are sucking vigorously.

Most mothers who decide to breast feed find the experience rewarding. Although involving extra work and some temporary discomfort at first, they find it very satisfying to finally establish a healthy nursing baby on the breast. It is also more convenient as there are no bottles to sterilize or feeds to prepare.

The nursing staff realize the importance of breast feeding and will be enthusiastic to help you. Another very important source of help is La Leche League International; they publish excellent literature and counsellors are available who have practical experience with the difficulties encountered in successful breast feeding.

Not every woman wishes to breast feed; inevitably there will be some mothers who either decide not to attempt breast feeding or else stop if they feel the problems are too great. If you decide to artificially feed your baby, alternative food preparations are available.

What does breast feeding of a premature baby entail?

1 Expressing the colostrum and later the breast milk while in hospital, either by hand or using some form of breast pump. This colostrum or milk is delivered regularly to the special nursery. It is often given without sterilization, but only to your own baby. The breasts produce very small amounts of colostrum until the 'milk comes in' on the third or fourth day.

2 At home, regular expressions of milk are required at least five times each twenty-four hours. The milk is kept scrupulously clean and is refrigerated.

3 Every day, the previous twenty-four hours expression of milk is delivered to the special nursery. The mother, or any willing person can deliver the milk which should be kept cool during transport to the hospital.

4 If it is not possible to deliver the milk each day, ask about deep freezing the milk and making less frequent trips to the hospital. Hospitals have their own rules and guidelines for you to follow.

5 As soon as the staff consider the baby may be ready to suck, one feed daily at the breast is tried; at first the baby will not suck

well, but will gradually improve over the next two or three weeks. As described in Chapter 3, this skin contact phase of establishing baby at mother's breast is satisfying for mother and baby, even if the baby gets very little milk.

6 Close to the time of going home, the mother will usually need to come into the hospital for at least two feeds daily and maybe more.

7 Frequently, mothers are able to express only enough milk to partly meet their baby's needs whilst he is in hospital. However, once she has the additional stimulation of the baby sucking directly on the breast, the supply usually improves and the amount increases to meet the baby's needs.

How to establish a good supply of milk

Under normal conditions, a hungry baby supplies two of the important factors needed to establish a good supply of breast milk, namely nervous stimulation from suckling and frequent, complete emptying of the breasts. A confident relaxed attitude on the part of the mother and staff is also important. If your baby is premature, at first you will not have the stimulation because your baby is not able to suck vigorously; however, expressing the milk frequently will empty the breasts and can partly imitate the stimulation that sucking would provide. For the first two or three days only a small amount of colostrum is produced; then the 'milk comes in' and quite a large amount of milk can be expressed.

As the milk is made it flows to a reservoir just behind the nipple. When a baby sucks at the breast, the milk is expressed by the pressure of the jaws on the outer edges of the areola (or brown part). This can be imitated by expressing the milk by hand, using finger and thumb on opposite sides of the breast. It is important for you to find the correct place to express yourself as all breasts are slightly different. It is also important that you do not make yourself sore. To prevent sore patches, the finger and thumb used to express must remain in one place, opening and closing, not moving them up and down the breast.

Hand pumps and electric pumps are available and can be a great help to some mothers — others find that expressing is quicker and more comfortable by hand. All methods have their place and you may have to try all three to find the best method for you. Producing breast milk is affected by emotion; realizing that the effort to get the milk is worthwhile and thinking nobody but you can produce the very best for your baby will help. Many mothers find that thinking about her baby while expressing increases the flow of milk.

Do not be discouraged if after the first few weeks the supply is diminishing. With determination and hard work at expressing, it is easy to increase the supply when it is time for the baby to come to you. If you are not producing the required amount of milk, then increase the frequency of expressing during the day, expressing at night only if you feel uncomfortable. As your breasts will replace the milk expressed in approximately half to one hour, the frequency with which you express at intervals during the day is important in increasing the supply rather than the period spent at any one time. It is a good guide to stop expressing when the milk comes in drops, rather than spurts. Approximately five to ten minutes every two to three hours will build up the supply.

Demand feeding your premature baby starts when he has learned to suck well and wakes up hungry. This usually happens at about his expected date of birth (forty weeks). When you go home your paediatrician will usually advise you to keep your baby on demand feeding, feeding him whenever he wakes and is hungry. At first this may be every one to two hours until your milk supply builds up. It is usually better to restrict each time at the breast to no longer than half-an-hour.

The information given in this chapter is brief, firstly because this may be all you want to know immediately after the birth of your premature baby and, secondly, because there are some excellent publications available for further reading. These include:

La Leche League International pamphlets (9616 Minneapolis Ave., P.O. Box 1209, Franklin Park, IL 60131-8209):

Breastfeeding Your Premature Baby
Mothering Multiples
Medications for the Nursing Mother
Establishing Your Milk Supply
Working and Nursing

CHAPTER 5

Parents' feelings after the birth of a premature baby

For most parents the birth of a premature baby is a very distressing experience and one for which they usually are unprepared. The hospital staff realize that not only are they responsible for the medical care of the baby but also for the well-being of the parents whose feelings during this crisis are extremely important. The professionals, doctors, nurses, social workers and others, can often be a great help; also other parents who have shared your experience may be invaluable. As parents you are entitled to assistance. No two families have exactly similar needs and the hospital staff will certainly try to give you what you want and at the time you feel you are ready. In other words, you should move at your own pace.

It is not our intention to tell you how you should feel and react. No two people deal with a difficulty in precisely the same fashion. People's own personal experiences and perceptions can contribute to different reactions to a seemingly similar event. Nevertheless, there are some general reactions, some of which mothers and fathers of premature babies will recognize in themselves. It is usually a comfort to realize that your thoughts, feelings and worries have been experienced by others; even more importantly, that in time these worries will resolve. There are many ways of working through these feelings. Talking about worries does help and it is our aim to stimulate you to discuss your anxieties with sympathetic health care professionals. It can also be helpful to speak with parents who have had similar experiences.

Emotional reactions in a pregnancy that goes to term

During pregnancy, parents often build up a rather idealized mental picture of the baby they are expecting to be born. The process develops through pregnancy and at term the most likely picture will include a chubby, healthy strong infant, an object of pride who will be prettily dressed, a pleasure to feed and care for, perhaps holding promise for a future encompassing some of those things that parents have not been able to achieve. These ideas and the mental picture of the baby evolve gradually and the mother forms a strong emotional attachment to this expected child.

Definite and positive expectations for the entire birth experience are established, including participation of the partner and sometimes family and friends. Towards the expected day, there is a general impatience to end the discomforts and restrictions imposed by pregnancy. Some parents have a less positive reaction with considerable apprehension that the baby will be abnormal in some way; only the birth of a healthy baby will resolve this nagging worry. The birth of a premature baby interferes with these reactions in many ways.

First images and reactions

To many parents the very premature baby at birth does not look attractive. Many parents initially say 'isn't she beautiful' or something else complimentary because they wish to please the nursing staff or want to appear 'normal' parents. Many are not ready to face their own feelings of shock and disbelief. Sooner or later many volunteer that they were shocked and appalled when they first saw their baby. They often liken the baby to an animal or bird. 'She looked like a skinned rabbit and I thought, "How horrid — a tiny featherless bird tossed out of his nest!".

Another mother told us later, 'I would not look at her, I fixed my eyes just beyond her so nobody knew how I felt'.

Mixed feelings are common. On the one hand parents want to love their baby, but on the other hand are afraid, either because of his appearance or because they fear to invest their love in case he dies and then the hurt would be worse.

Gradually parents cope with these feelings and their perceptions change. Later a mother said, 'I began to know his face, his expression, it was as if I had always known him'. So by six weeks the appearance of baby is far more acceptable — rather spindly legs, a biggish head, always sleeping, but to most parents a thing of beauty.

However, babies born twelve weeks before the expected date look so different from the full term infant that it is hard to visualize such a tiny, feeble, hairy, red scrap of humanity ever going to school, playing football or one day becoming a mother or father. The initial doubts for the future are perfectly natural. When you understand this, you will begin to accept your baby as an individual and a special member of the family.

The staff of a special care nursery understand this initial shock and disappointment so it is not necessary to hide these feelings.

The birth and surrounding events

The birth of a healthy baby at term is usually an extremely happy time for both the mother and father. With proper preparation of the mother during pregnancy, sympathetic and skilful care during labour and the husband very frequently present at the birth, the first contact with baby is a time of great joy and fulfilment. Almost immediately the mother is able to feed, fondle, touch and admire her offspring so that she and her baby remain as one close unit, even though they are now physically separate individuals.

In the usual situation, the mother can expect a normal labour, with a minimum of fuss, equipment and concern from the delivery room staff. Once the baby is born, the immediate crying of the babe and the opportunity to look at and hold the infant confirms that all is well. In contrast, the mother of the premature infant has not experienced the 'winding down' period when she physically and mentally prepares for the coming birth. She does not have the experience of being ready for labour, it simply arrives like an unwelcome visitor. Once in the labour ward the major emphasis is on giving the baby the best possible chance of living. This experience of labour does not coincide with mother's expectations. Because drugs given to the mother during labour may make the premature baby sluggish at birth, they are given less liberally than usual, therefore the mother may experience more discomfort. To protect the premature baby from injury, a forceps delivery is often used and an episiotomy ('stitches') is also frequently necessary for the same reason. All these measures are taken to **protect** the baby from injury.

It is usual to have a paediatrician or specially trained nurse at the delivery, so that the necessary care for baby can commence right away. The very premature baby rarely cries immediately and he is quickly placed in a warm place where oxygen and other simple treatment is given. It is often several minutes before the baby can be shown to the mother and unrestricted contact is usually not possible.

There is now rather a hurry to move the baby to the special care nursery so that he does not get cold. It is not possible to undress the baby for the mother to inspect him and certainly no possibility of suckling at the breast.

So far, there has been very little possibility for mother and baby to experience the togetherness as was described for the term baby.

Feelings of guilt, grief, sadness and loss

(a) **Loss of normal labour**
Many mothers feel deprived because they missed the experience of a normal labour. One said, 'It was supposed to be the great event — to me it was just a nightmare; I hoped I'd wake and find it hadn't happened'. Others are disturbed and confused, being unable to identify their feelings: 'It was over. I was lost. I wondered if I'd had a baby at all.'

Because the labour was early and their bodies had not behaved in the normal way some women experience feelings of guilt and failure. They suspect that in some way they have caused the labour to be early, and they feel failure because their bodies have not performed up to expectations.

(b) **Loss of the perfect baby**
Many feel that the perfect baby they have built in their imagination is lost, replaced by an imperfect substitute.

(c) **Loss of the baby to the special care unit**
The removal of the baby to a special care unit is a separation that most mothers find hard to endure. No matter how soon and how often the nursery is visited, this loss may remain.

(d) **Loss of control**
For many the loss of control of the circumstances of birth are often deeply resented; again an expectation that is unfulfilled, as most mothers look forward to participating in the process. The hospital and attendants may be perceived as impersonal and indifferent, and unnecessarily interfering.

(e) **Loss of part of self**
Some mothers feel that they are losing a part of themselves, that the baby is not ready to leave the womb until the expected day of delivery.

Grief

The feelings we have described may lead to grief. Some parents grieve the loss of what might have been a normal joyous event, and a normal healthy infant. Others grieve, almost in preparation for the infant's death. This is especially likely to happen if parents are initially given an unnecessarily gloomy forecast of their baby's chances of survival.

Through frank expression of feeling and sharing with the partner, and through staff who are trained to help and through the help of other mothers, most parents are able to traverse this painful phase and grow to optimism and confidence in themselves and their baby.

Anger and depression

Anger is another common feeling. 'Why should this happen to us?' This anger often gives way to depression. It is a normal part of grief which some mothers and fathers naturally express in frequent outbursts of tears. Others who are depressed quietly withdraw. Grief and depression last for varying periods, but often continue long after the premature baby is out of danger.

Many mothers describe the return of waves of anger or depression for many weeks, again long after there is any medical anxiety for the babies.

Within this framework of loss and grief there are some other commonly expressed reactions.

Feelings of unreality

'I don't feel I have a baby' and 'I look at her and feel she is not mine' are very frequent statements of mothers in the first few days. These impressions are especially strong if the birth was by Caesarean section under a general anaesthetic. Mothers with pre-eclampsia (kidney trouble) often require large amounts of sedatives around the time of birth and many are drowsy for a few days, and may be confused and unable to go to the nursery to see their baby. In these circumstances the instant colour photograph of her baby, available in many nurseries, helps a little. When regular visiting is possible, touching and assisting with baby care helps to overcome these feelings of unreality, doubt and disbelief. It is normal to have these feelings and to take time to accept the baby.

Feelings of jealousy

Mothers sometimes resent the caretakers or others who have more contact with the baby. One mother said, 'I envy the intensive care staff; they are with her all the time; I feel useless, as if they have taken her away from me.' They may also feel resentful of other mothers in their wards or visiting friends with healthy children.

Sleeplessness and other symptoms

Many parents find their normal sleep pattern disturbed. They may have difficulty getting off to sleep or waken during the night with a feeling of anxiety which sometimes can only be relieved by telephoning the nursery to reassure themselves that there is no reason for this sudden panic. This is also a time when parents find themselves unable to make decisions, lack concentration or are overwhelmingly tired.

Visiting the Intensive Care Nursery

In the Intensive Care Nursery infants are usually critically ill and the overwhelming impression is of busy staff and a confusion of equipment. The technology and the machines may be quite frightening to some parents.

For many, this will be their first direct experience of severe illness. Lack of privacy in which to see their baby and shed some quiet tears may be very distressing. Few parents will be prepared

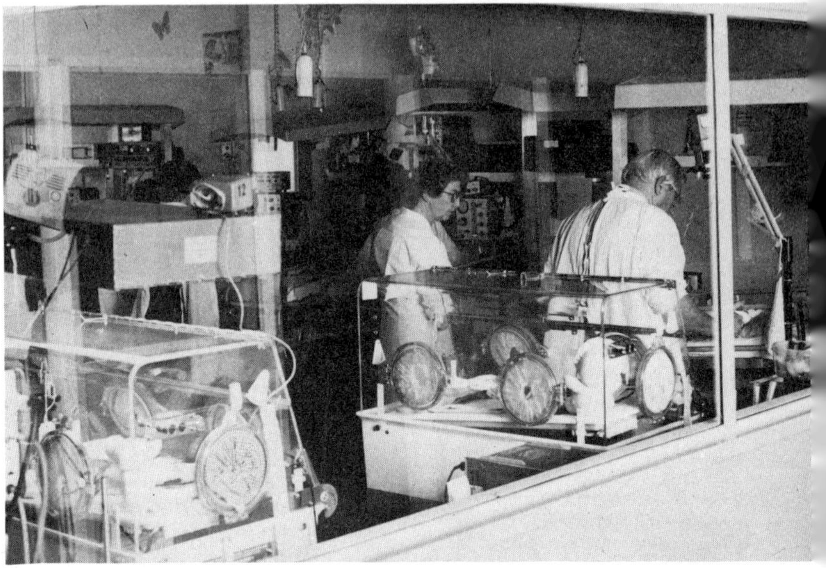

A look through the window into the intensive care unit. The room looks cluttered and may seem impersonal. When you get inside to see your baby you will be made to feel welcome and equipment will become familiar to you; things you see surrounding your baby will be explained.

for such unnerving experiences. The whole area may seem unreal, rather like a scene from science fiction. Under these circumstances, the parents often feel superfluous, helpless intruders. The baby may look so fragile that it is hard to believe that he can be handled.

The staff in such a unit are not only experts in the care of these babies, they also appreciate that you, as parents, will be alarmed, apprehensive and uncertain in this strange environment and that this baby belongs to **you**, not the nursing or medical staff. Initially, the environment of the intensive care unit will be strange, but as you get to know the doctors and nurses, you will become comfortable there. When in the nursery, be ready to ask questions about your baby and all aspects related to his care.

The growth of attachment (bonding)

Parents usually develop a strong emotional attachment to their children, and very early in life a baby comes to appreciate that parents are the special individuals who give care and love. In recent years the word 'bonding' has been used to describe this tie or attachment between members of the family unit; the word 'bonding' is new, but the attachment and protection of the young is not.

Parents who read about bonding may get the mistaken idea that attachment between mother and baby happens in a dramatic way immediately after birth. This is not so, and although there are many for whom the feeling is immediate, there are many in whom this feeling develops over time. Some fathers find this attachment does not begin until the baby smiles at them and many mothers do not feel maternal towards their babies until they have them home and are fully responsible for their every need.

Medical care and physical problems of prematurity make the normal process of attachment more difficult. The intimate and intensely private relationship which involves holding, cuddling and gazing at each other is not possible for mother and baby. In other words, the baby cannot stimulate the mother's response in the same way as the normal healthy full-term infant does. However, visiting the baby in the nursery as soon as possible, touching and talking to the baby in the incubator and participating in his care as he grows will all help attachment to develop.

Touching your baby and helping with care

Some parents have no difficulty in approaching their small baby, touching the hand or stroking the forehead, but many will take a few days before they can do this comfortably if at all. This should not be forced or hurried. It is something you do at your own pace. This first touching and fondling is usually a highly emotional experience, with the mixed feelings of intense pleasure and fear that touching may cause harm. Parents learn quite soon that, far from causing damage, both parents and their baby get great benefit from these visits. Touching and talking to the baby help to develop that special attachment or bond between mother and child that was disrupted by the necessary separation after the birth. For the extremely sick or small baby, there is not a huge amount that the parent can do to help physically, but the nurses will involve you whenever it is possible. At this stage simply being there will help you to know your baby and develop affectionate ties. Gradually, as the baby becomes bigger and stronger, you will be able to help more with his care. In the early stages, the mother's main contribution is to touch the baby and, if you aim to breast feed, to express breast milk and establish a good supply for later on.

As parents are able to take a greater part in their baby's care, and at a pace they feel comfortable, attachment and parental love **will grow naturally**.

Restriction of visiting

Most units encourage parents to visit as frequently as they wish and at any time. Often there are some restrictions concerning the number of visitors who may come into the nursery because there is not sufficient room for large numbers of people. Overcrowding would make it impossible to give the high standard of care these babies require. Relatives and friends may certainly come to see your baby at a distance. In some hospitals, other family members are also able to come into the nursery if there is sufficient room. Ask for the guidelines of the particular hospital where your baby is being cared for.

Ideally, visiting special care units should be possible at any time. A little thought shows that certain times will be less convenient for the staff and therefore parents will receive less attention and information. Most nurseries are extremely busy at the beginning of the working day when doctors and nurses are planning the day's changes in treatment and arranging x-rays and a variety of blood tests. The early afternoon when the early shift of nursing staff hands over to the next group of nurses may also be a busy time. Finally, in special care nurseries there are emergencies when nurses and doctors are so fully occupied with care of a baby that it is not possible to answer the visiting parents' questions right at that moment. If you are unexpectedly left waiting outside the nursery, this is usually the reason. Parents often assume that the emergency concerns their own baby and worry unnecessarily. Ask and put your mind at ease!

On the first day or so, you will probably only have eyes for your own baby, but gradually you will begin to see other premature infants and meet their parents. It is often helpful to see another infant smaller and 'sicker' than yours, and parents of babies who are older than yours can also help you. However, nursery staff discourage the parent who does a 'daily ward round' of the nursery asking for a progress report on each patient. Apart from the time involved, each baby's progress is a completely confidential matter between individual parents and staff.

In these first few days, an ever present question is: 'will our baby survive?' A book like this can only answer the question in general terms, but the doctors and nurses are able to give you a more accurate prediction. Certainly a few premature babies still die, but in a modern intensive care nursery this is unusual and the general climate is one of well-founded optimism.

Should a birth notice go in the paper?

The birth notice in the paper is an individual decision. Like most other decisions, it is best that both parents talk this over. If the baby is very small or extremely sick, most parents decide to defer the birth notice, at least until the mother has gone home. If the medical situation is less serious, a birth notice may be considered that includes the words 'born prematurely' which is a kindness and a gentle caution to your friends. If parents decide that no birth notice is to be placed in the paper the husband has an important role as close friends should be encouraged to write to the mother in hospital or, better still, to visit. Flowers are so much a part of the celebration of a birth that friends and relatives should be told that it is a good idea to send them. Little gifts for the baby also carry a message of hope for most mothers.

Naming your baby

As soon as both parents feel they are ready it is a good idea to decide on the name that will suit your baby. Make sure that it is written on your baby's cot or incubator. Naming helps to make the baby a real individual for you and the nursery staff also find that a given name helps to make the nursery more friendly.

Sometimes you may find yourself pressured to make a decision on names. Our advice is to wait until you are ready. Although you are legally required to register your baby's birth, there is no hurry to do this.

How long will the danger period last?

Mercifully for many parents, the critical period is over in a few days and the doctors are then confident that all will go well.

For other parents this time of waiting may be very long. With improvements in the technology of intensive care, extremely premature babies now frequently survive, but only with the help of a ventilator to support life for days or even weeks. This can be an agonizing time with periods of gradual improvement. An unexpected complication may bring back all the recent anxieties and fears that parents believed were past. Sometimes days and even weeks go by with so little improvement that parents despair of their baby ever going home. Weight gains or oxygen concentrations become a matter of great excitement if the news is favourable, or of depression if parents' goals and expectations are not realized. The staff find it hard too, for they also hope for a faster improvement and are frustrated and disappointed when this does not happen.

Tension between parents

Parents who have a warm, loving relationship usually provide help, support and comfort to each other during a long period of anxiety or at times when their baby has setbacks. Finally, their relationship is likely to be enriched by their shared experience. It would be surprising if this mutual help and support always went smoothly. Parents often readjust to their anxieties at different rates or may cope with anxiety in different ways. This may cause temporary misunderstandings; for example, where a husband whose anxiety has eased, constantly tells his wife not to worry. The mother may continue to worry and be angry with him for not understanding her concern.

Sometimes one parent, either mother or father, tries to take all the worry in order to spare the other. Such consideration is undoubtedly well motivated, but in almost every situation, bad news as well as good news is better shared. It is not uncommon for one partner to be so stressed and exhausted that he or she feels unable to cope with any additional emotional demand that their partner or relatives may be making. Because it takes all of one parent's emotional resources to cope with him or herself, it may be hard, or even impossible, to help the other partner. Occasionally one or both parents may be so anxious and depressed that communication between them is almost impossible. Some intensive care units have a social worker available to counsel parents who are experiencing these difficulties. If this service is not available at your hospital ask your paediatrician where such professional help may be obtained.

Feelings about death

Not all parents want the baby to live and some who were initially enthusiastic gradually or suddenly wish for their baby's death. This is a thought that many people experience but are unwilling to put into words because it sounds too callous or unnatural, or because it would seem they were lacking in gratitude to the staff who have cared for baby. Our advice is to talk this through. Sometimes it is a nurse that will share this confidence, at other times the doctor or social worker, but they will **not** be shocked by this attitude. There are many reasons for these negative feelings. Parents are concerned that the baby is suffering pain, although usually this is not so. Possibly the pregnancy was initially unwanted, or maybe friends or relatives have been telling the parents about premature babies who did not grow up normally. Sometimes there is financial concern. On the other hand, these feelings may be part of a normal **grieving process** and will not persist.

These, or any other worries, are better shared with a professional person who usually can help you through these negative feelings to a new perspective. Most intensive care staff are very sensitive to the spoken and unspoken feelings of parents. In the case of an infant with a clearly hopeless outlook for the future the use of life-support measures is often tactfully and unobtrusively withheld. Your doctor cannot participate in euthanasia, but in relation to such cases, before some treatment decisions are made, it is vital for the staff to know how you really feel.

Changing feelings as the baby grows

Even the most sensible, well informed parents dealing with sympathetic, relaxed and exceptionally helpful nursery staff are unlikely to be able to avoid all the pitfalls and anxieties described. However, having an awareness of these factors, and also being able to share them, should reduce the trauma and baby's growth and progress will provide the source of optimism.

A milestone is reached on the day when baby is well enough to come out of the incubator to be cuddled by both father and mother. Next follows the initiation into bottle feeding and then putting the baby to the breast. Another big step is the demonstration in bathing when even the experienced mother may be distressed at the small size of the baby and worry that he will become cold or be dropped when he is slippery and wet. The nurse, carrying out this important part of mothercraft teaching will understand these worries, and she should welcome practical questions.

Building confidence

In spite of what many people believe, mothering is not a natural ability that women possess. Therefore, women do not take on this role with the ease and confidence that is sometimes unreasonably expected of them. Confidence and competence come with practice and those feelings of self-esteem, which are built up by success. The mother of the premature infant may have her self-esteem and confidence disrupted by the circumstances of the birth. Taking over the role of caring for an infant who was visibly so small and fragile is quite a big step. She needs a great deal of help and encouragement from the nursery staff and later, at home, from her family. Whilst she is learning the practical details of how to care for baby and building up this feeling, she should be prepared to ask for help.

Final preparation for taking the baby home

Sometimes the final preparation of mother and baby for the major move home is not well managed. A sudden increase in admission of sick babies may mean that relatively healthy ones need to be 'pushed out' as soon as possible. If you are not fully confident of your ability to handle the baby, you may need extra help. Ask your paediatrician or the hospital staff to recommend a nurse or an infant care helper who can come to your home.

Once the premature baby has been home for a few weeks, the parents usually have achieved confidence in their own ability and are beginning to thoroughly enjoy the baby, watching him grow and smile, laugh and quickly mature into a real personality.

CHAPTER 6 Family and friends: how can they help?

Grandparents and close friends are sometimes uncertain how to be of help. It is important for them to understand that giving birth to a premature baby is a very upsetting crisis for parents. It will be much easier if they understand the parents' needs and feelings, so that they can be of positive assistance and avoid advice and comments that unintentionally upset the parents.

It must be realized that the parents may be disorganized and distraught. This state of affairs may go on for months; even after all the medical worries are over and the baby is doing well at home, some parents are still having some difficulties in coping. During this time they are in very special need of love, support, and acceptance. They are specially vulnerable to criticism and bad advice and innocent remarks can be misinterpreted. All these things may have long-lasting ill effects. Sometimes a sympathetic, well-intentioned relative will say 'do not mind too much if she dies, you can always have another baby later'. Such advice is deeply resented and can be taken to mean that the baby has little or no value. Parents at this vulnerable and sensitive time frequently find: 'Don't worry, you will soon have him home' very distressing. As one mother said, 'I have every reason to worry, and I know he won't come home for weeks. To be told not to worry makes me mad'. It requires great patience and understanding to bear with this often slow recovery of parents from the experiences surrounding the birth of a premature, sick baby.

If relatives and friends would like to know more about how the parents may be feeling, they should also read Chapter 5.

The birth of a baby is usually an occasion of great pleasure and excitement, not only for the parents but for the other children, grandparents and friends. The mother receives cards, gifts and flowers. Visitors come to admire the new baby. The proud father receives the congratulations of work mates and friends and plans for the future turn over in his mind. Birth notices go in the paper; the debate on names has to be resolved. Admittedly this ideal situation rarely goes quite smoothly, but usually this is a very happy, fulfilling time for the parents.

However, for the parents and close relatives of an infant born prematurely, things may be very different. Many of the parents feel sad, cheated and resentful because so many of the anticipated pleasures surrounding a normal birth are not fulfilled. There are some practical ways in which relatives and close friends **can** help without being intrusive or aggravating the distress of parents.

The maternity hospital room without flowers and cards is depressing. The thoughtful husband can make sure that close friends and relatives take appropriate, early action. Wording in cards, such as 'thinking of you' or 'get well' may be more suitable than congratulations. If no birth notice is placed in the paper, close friends should be encouraged to write to the mother in hospital if they cannot visit. These letters may be more difficult to write but they are extraordinarily helpful to the recipient in a time of crisis. The giving of small presents for the infant tells the mother that her relatives and friends believe that the baby does have a chance of living — and, of course, the majority of premature babies do go home.

Hospital can be a particularly painful place to stay for the mother of a sick, premature baby. She is often unavoidably separated for much of the day from her baby in the nursery. Meeting other mothers caring for their babies may be an emotionally painful and recurrent experience. The routine of meals, visitors, expressing the breast milk and visiting her baby which fill the day can often leave a mother surprisingly exhausted, even though she is normally active and busy. Unrestricted visiting of husband and close relatives is now the policy in most hospitals, so if the mother feels she can cope with visitors why not try to visit as frequently as possible.

Visiting the premature baby

Most parents are pleased to allow grandparents and other relatives and friends to go to the special care nursery to see the new member of the family, but sometimes the baby is so small and surrounded by so much equipment that the first sight may be quite a shock. Visitors are not alone in this reaction, for often parents describe their first impression of their baby with such unfavourable similes as 'like a wrinkled little old man' or 'a rabbit'. However, it should be realized that while parents may sometimes allow themselves such expressions they are often very hurt when others make similar observations.

Mothers and fathers of premature babies take time to adjust to the unexpected appearance of premature babies. Relatives and friends also will find their original expectations of a big, vigorous, full-term infant must change. They too adjust in time. Soon the small, initially less attractive, premature baby will be a real person whom they can accept and love.

Grandparents of a premature baby, with their longer experience of the world than their own children, are often very worried that the baby may grow to be intellectually retarded or physically handicapped. Possibly they or their friends had this experience years ago when the outlook for a premature baby was not nearly as hopeful as today. It is important to realize that most small babies cared for in special nurseries grow up and succeed at school just like other children.

Occasionally, grandparents of babies born very early believe it is helpful to prepare their children for the premature baby's death. Here again expectations have changed dramatically. Twenty years ago, if a baby was born 12 weeks early, less than one in every ten had a hope of survival. Nowadays, one expects about eight in every ten to eventually go home.

However, grandparents are often an important influence at this time and can be of enormous positive benefit to the parents of a premature baby. One of their most important roles is to be available to listen when the parents are ready to talk about their worries. They can also provide practical help by assisting with other children in the family, minding them while the mother visits her baby, or perhaps helping with transport. When the baby goes home, the tactful grandparent is able to provide encouragement and help without flaunting her experience and 'taking over' the care of the baby.

The other children at home

In the anxiety for the premature baby and his parents any other children at home should not be forgotten. They too are part of the family and probably will be upset. Most parents prepare the older children for the homecoming of a term baby. With a premature birth the other children are usually quite unprepared either for their mother's sudden disappearance to hospital for the birth of the baby or, later, the frequent trips to visit the new baby in hospital. The anxiety of parents is usually sensed by children even if not put into words.

Although hospital routines vary, it is not always possible for the premature baby to be cuddled by older children; however, they can nearly always see their new brother or sister. Provided parents are present and there is not too much equipment around, small children react to a premature baby with interest and apparently without much anxiety. If the experience is upsetting to a small child, lack of interest in the new baby or moving away are important hints to adults that the child does not want to be pushed further. Allow the child to move at his own pace towards acceptance of the new baby. It is necessary to explain, within the children's comprehension, the reasons for leaving the baby in hospital for a time.

Children who share in the family distress are likely to 'behave badly' and can sometimes be a great trial just when the family needs no more problems. Food refusal, temper-tantrums, waking at night, clinging to the parents, crying, wetting the bed and aggressive or destructive behaviour are just some of the troubles that may develop. This regression to the behaviour of a younger child needs to be understood by the adults for what it really is — a child's method of dealing with stress, insecurity and anxiety. Understanding, patience and tolerance rather than discipline or punishment usually help the child to return to normal, otherwise professional advice should be obtained.

Whenever possible, the other children should be at home rather than staying with relatives when the premature baby finally leaves hospital. They generally need little encouragement to gently touch or kiss the new brother or sister and 'help' with the care at home. Children should not feel excluded and in any way unwanted or a nuisance at this time.

Soon he'll be playing with Teddy.

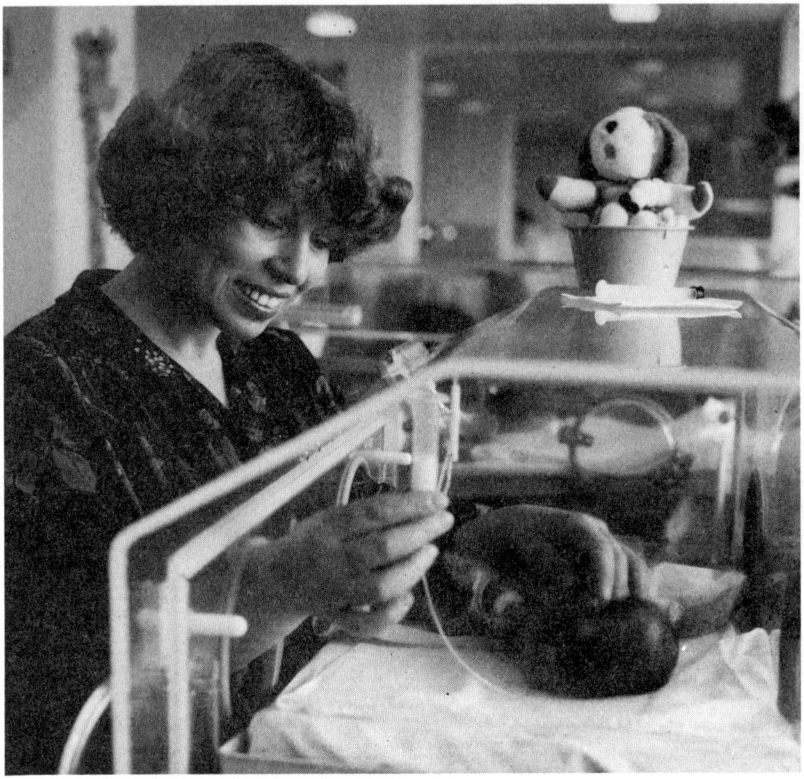

CHAPTER 7 Your premature baby comes home at last

Parents of both premature and term babies eagerly await the pleasure of the homecoming, but there is often a little anxiety too. For the first time, parents have the full responsibility for the care of the new baby and it may take a little time to become fully confident and comfortable.

Regular visits to your baby in hospital will have prepared you for feeding, changing diapers and bathing your baby. In hospital you will have learned a great deal about your baby's signals showing hunger, discomfort and boredom; you will know how to meet these needs with either feeding, changing or comforting and talking to your baby. In the first few days at home you will quickly become even better in anticipating or meeting his needs and it becomes more and more obvious that small babies have their own distinctive personalities and that they can communicate their needs to parents.

Where to get help and advice

Some premature babies need to be fed very frequently at home, but otherwise the physical care is usually no more demanding than that of any other new baby. However, there will be times when the new parents will need reassurance that they are doing everything correctly or will require advice on some aspect of baby care. This help can be found from a number of sources:

(a) **The Neonatal Intensive Care Unit.** Particularly in the first few days after leaving hospital, a telephone call to the Neonatal Intensive Care Unit will usually allow you to talk to a nurse who knows you and your baby.

(b) **Family Doctor, Paediatrician or Hospital.** You may feel it is a good idea to take your baby to a doctor for examination if you are really worried. A paediatrician or a neonatologist – a paediatrician who specializes in premature and high-risk newborns – may be more experienced in your baby's special needs than a general practitioner.

(c) **La Leche League International.** As already mentioned, their counsellors are available to help in matters relating to difficulties with

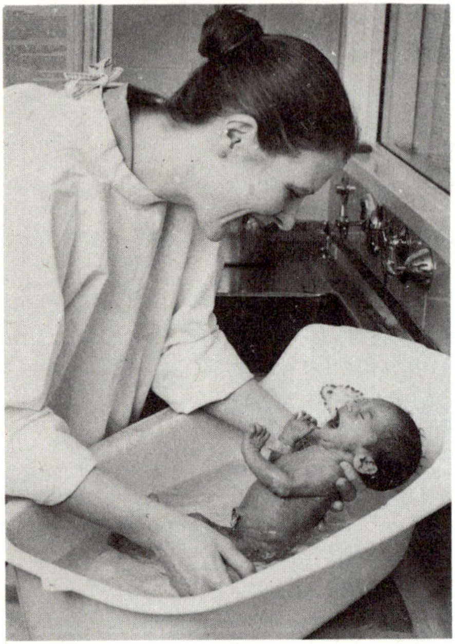

A first bath for Jessica who is not too sure about enjoying it. Her mother has her safely held and a staff member is at hand if help is needed.

breast feeding. In most states a twenty-four hour telephone number is available.

(d) **Relatives and friends.** Those who have reared their own children frequently have a lot of practical experience with the 'minor' problems of newborn babies that are not 'minor' to anxious parents. While the reassurance of friends is sometimes useful, advice from a variety of friends and relatives is likely to be conflicting, so if in real doubt, consult one of the professionals.

(e) **Premature parents' support groups and clubs** are very helpful. Contact Parents of Premature and High-Risk Infants International, Inc. (33 W. 42nd St., New York, NY 10036) for the group closest to you.

Care of your baby at home

The physical care of the premature baby when he comes home and the necessary preparation and requirements are essentially those needed for any healthy newborn baby. Unless you have been told otherwise by your paediatrician, your baby should be treated just like any other that leaves the maternity hospital for he is now mature, able to feed and is having no special trouble keeping warm.

If you have prepared a separate nursery, there is no reason why he should not occupy this immediately; for convenience at night you may wish to keep the bassinette at your bedside so that night feeds are a little easier. At home he will need about the same amount of clothing as used at the end of his stay in hospital. It is not necessary to warm the bedroom unless the house is exceptionally cold or you have been instructed otherwise. Hot water bottles and temperature taking, a feature of the hospital, will not be needed any more. A warm room for the bath is a kindness. For the first two weeks, a quick bath on alternate days is usually sufficient. Like so many mothers of term babies you may still be a little worried about bathing your baby; the presence of the father or an experienced relative or friend may help to establish confidence.

Initially the premature baby is fed at intervals throughout the twenty-four hours of the day. Shortly before going home, feedings are usually changed to approximately every four hours and the baby is encouraged to sleep after the 10.00 p.m. feed until 6.00 o'clock next morning. Sometimes this routine may not be well established and you may find when you take baby home that he wakes at night and that he is demanding his feeds at intervals of less than four hours.

If baby is fully breast fed, settling well after feeds and gaining weight you should not worry at all about the volume of milk he is obtaining. Quite often, the baby goes home partly breast fed, but still taking a little at each feed from a bottle. With demand feeding your milk supply will usually improve, while bottle feeding will decrease. If the infant has a regular night feeding, the mother may have an occasional rest if father feels sufficiently confident to give expressed breast milk or formula.

If the baby is on a bottle, the hospital will have provided details of the preparation of the formula and an indication of the volume that is likely to be taken. It is very important to prepare the formula exactly as instructed. If the volume of the feed is not great enough to satisfy your baby, do not add extra water. Make up a larger volume of formula. If you are not sure of quantities, ask your paediatrician. It is important to measure quantities exactly as you were shown in hospital and **not** to add a 'little' extra milk powder to make the baby grow more quickly. If baby is hungry, you give a bigger volume of the same strength formula. The average infant when leaving hospital needs about 90-120 ml (3-4 ounces) at each feeding but many demand more; it is safe and proper to feed to the baby's appetite. The amount taken from a bottle often varies greatly from feed to feed. If your baby takes less than 60 ml (2 ounces) for several consecutive feeds, you should consult your doctor. An occasional poor feed by itself is no cause for worry. Vomiting of small amounts after feeds is extremely common but large persistent vomiting needs to be reported.

Within a week of taking baby home, he should be weighed for this confirms that feedings are going well. In the first week, a gain of 100 g (about 3 ounces) is usual and thereafter weight gains are often greater. Regular visits to your paediatrician are very important. You will have a host of questions to ask over the next few months and regular checking of weight gains **and** advice on diet and commencement of the immunization programme will all be arranged.

Newborn Noises. If this is your first baby you may be surprised by some of the peculiar noises made by healthy babies at home, especially at night when all is quiet. Slight blockage of the nose and sneezing, which are almost always noted, do not indicate that baby has a cold. Little grunts and whimpers during sleep are common. The normal baby always passes wind from the bowel and this does not mean that you have not 'brought up the wind' correctly. Hiccoughs are very common and are not an indication that the infant has been fed incorrectly.

Baby's cry. Often you will be able to identify the cause. Hunger, boredom, a wet or dirty diaper, being over-clothed or wrapped up too tightly may all make a baby protest in the only effective way known to him. It is common for babies to have one crying, wakeful period, often around 6.00 p.m., a time at which maximum domestic disruption may be caused. The mother may find that even after making the baby as comfortable as possible he continues to cry for a while. It is important not to become too anxious about this but realize that it is normal behaviour.

The baby with colic

Many babies, both full term and premature, at times display difficult behaviour which may be described as 'colic', 'hyperactivity' or 'wind'. They tend to sleep for short periods, often lying awake looking about for longer periods than is expected of a small baby. They may cry for long periods of time for no apparent reason. This behaviour is seen in 20 per cent of normal infants. Four facts need to be clearly understood:

- This behaviour is common
- The cause for this type of behaviour is not known with certainty, but it practically never has any serious basis
- The infant's behaviour can be greatly improved and parents can be reassured if their doctor sees the baby and gives them appropriate advice and maybe some medicine for the infant
- This behaviour is **not** caused by incorrect feeding technique

Restless behaviour of the type just described also occurs with some premature babies who have been home a few days. Possibly the activity, disturbances, lights and noises of a special care nursery have upset them more than the usual infant. It is important to see a doctor so that effective treatment can be given to calm the baby and authoritatively reassure the parents that there is no serious cause. There are strategies for coping with these restless babies, and your doctor will be able to advise you about these measures. Gentle massage and skin contact help some of these restless babies.

Growth and weight gains

Babies who are small because of premature delivery usually grow quite as well as those born at the expected date, although it may take a few months to make up for the rather poor growth in the first few weeks in hospital.

Babies who are small because they grow poorly in the womb (intrauterine growth retardation) sometimes have quite a different pattern. Their weight gains at home may be small and their appetite for milk may also be less than other infants; later on only tiny amounts of solids may be taken. Some growth retarded infants remain less than average size in later childhood. Whilst some of these children have a spurt of growth at puberty, many grow into smallish but normal adults. Often their size will be similar to that of their parents. If you are worried about this reduced rate of growth, discuss it with your doctor, but eventually you may have to accept the fact that it is this child's nature to be smaller than average.

Milestones of development and 'corrected age'

Because a baby is born prematurely, there is no speed-up in the development and function of the brain. A baby born at term has the first genuine meaningful smile at about six weeks of age. The baby who is born twelve weeks prematurely cannot be expected to smile properly until eighteen weeks after the actual birth — i.e. six weeks post-term. This 'corrected age' is therefore used in assessment of progress.

It must be emphasized that this apparent slowness in development is not a sign of retardation. It is invariable that eve premature baby starts his normal milestones of development from the due date, not the birth date. Relatives and friends who do not know this may easily upset parents of premature babies by remarking about small or apparently poor progress because they do not understand the need to make allowances for prematurity.

As each year goes by, this difference between actual and expected age becomes less and less important. At twenty-one years, it doesn't matter if you are only twenty years and nine months.

Physical health

As a rule, babies who were premature are as healthy as any oth child in the family. However there is a condition your doctor ma mention — **anaemia of prematurity**. This is not a cause for worr because it can be prevented if your premature baby has enough iron in the diet. Iron is essential for the body to make haemoglobin, the substance that gives blood its red colour. The baby who is born at full term has sufficient stored iron to last un solid foods are started, milk being relatively low in iron. The premature baby, however, has not had time to store the full quo of iron because of the premature birth, so extra iron is usually given to prevent anaemia. An infant with anaemia looks pale because he has fewer red cells in the blood and less of the red-coloured substance in the blood. Fortunately this anaemia is rarely severe, and it can be prevented by giving extra iron during the time baby is taking milk but no solids. Some milk formulae have enough iron added, but many breast fed and some bottle fed babies are ordered an iron-containing medicine.

The ex-premature baby is generally as healthy as his term counterpart. An exception will be the child who had **severe respiratory distress**, which needed a long period on the ventilator. These children may have bronchitis frequently in the first eighteen months of life. The doctor should therefore see these children fairly early with each 'cold' so that treatment shortens the attacks as much as possible. This tendency to bronchitis is expected to improve as the child gets older. If there is wheezing as well as cough, the doctor may call it bronchiolitis.

Immunization against diphtheria, whooping cough, tetanus, measles and poliomyelitis should be carried out just a little later than is the current practice in your community. It is especially important to get protection against infectious diseases early in infancy. Check with your doctor to be sure the timing of injections is right for your baby. Your doctor will give specific advice and would tell you if there was a special medical reason why your child should not be immunized against whooping cough or measles.

Feeding difficulties

Many completely healthy, normal babies born at full-term are difficult to feed at times. This often happens when the baby has a cold, is cutting teeth or the normal routine is upset in any way. Many healthy babies find it hard to accept solids when they are introduced and dislike new foods when they are first offered; many term babies take quite a long time to get used to taking foods which are at all lumpy. Premature babies behave like this too, so do not think this behaviour is abnormal.

If your baby is taking smaller breast or bottle feeds, it is particularly important not to force feed. You may feel happier to have your doctor check that all is well if the poor feeding lasts for long. With regard to solid foods, you will probably have less trouble if small amounts of solids are started relatively early; we would emphasize that the amounts should be small because your baby's needs will be largely satisfied by milk for the first few months. It is also important to realize that you should not wait until your baby has teeth before giving food with small lumps in it. Your paediatrician will give you specific advice on when to start solids and what to give.

Hearing problems

The majority of premature babies have hearing which is adequate for the development of normal speech. Severe deafness is now extremely rare.

It is usual for the paediatrician to arrange a hearing test towards the end of the first year of life.

All babies and small children may get ear infections, usually as a complication of a cold. Some children show they are in pain by crying and pulling at one or both ears. Usually the babies have a fever and often they are not drinking or are vomiting. Ear infections can only be diagnosed by your doctor who looks at the ear drums with a special instrument (auriscope). Ear infections require treatment which your doctor will arrange. Premature babies seem to get rather more ear infections than those born at term; if the ear infections do not respond to treatment given by your family doctor, referral to a specialist may be necessary.

S.I.D.S.

Most parents will have read in magazines or the newspapers that occasionally in the first year or so of life a healthy baby will die quite unexpectedly at home. This happens no matter how careful the parents are in their care of the infant and it is in no way their fault.

This sudden infant death syndrome (S.I.D.S.), or 'Cot Death', is an anxiety that parents of term and premature babies share and have to learn to live with. Possibly the risk is a little higher for the baby that was premature.

S.I.D.S. happens in about one in every 500 infants. It is not becoming more common and the extra publicity it has attracted in recent years is due to the fact that so many other reasons for losing an infant are now either preventable or are able to be successfully treated. For example, many malformations can now be completely corrected, and tuberculosis, measles, whooping cough and many other infections that once were killers can now be prevented or treated successfully with antibiotics.

At the turn of the century in developed countries, about one baby in every ten died in the first year of life. Nowadays, the risk of losing a baby from any cause, including S.I.D.S., is less than one in every hundred. Although nobody takes a baby home with a guarantee that all will go well, the prospects nowadays are far better than a few years ago.

The causes of S.I.D.S. are not fully understood. There is currently a great deal of research and hopefully we should get more information soon. If you are worried about S.I.D.S. you should certainly discuss this with your paediatrician.

Speech development

In children who were only slightly premature, there are usually no problems. Those babies who were extremely small may have some delay in commencing to use single words and a little later speech may sometimes be rather indistinct. This is a condition for which professional help should be sought. If there is any possibility of some reduction in hearing, tests should be carried out. Speech therapy may be needed. It must be stressed that these speech defects respond well to treatment; maybe the child will still be having some trouble at pre-school but when in the second or third year of school, speech should be normal.

Eye problems

Minor eye troubles are certainly far more common in children who were extremely premature. The only serious trouble — retrolental fibroplasia or R.L.F. — sometimes occurs despite the greatest care of the baby in the nursery; but in most nurseries, the very premature baby's eyes are regularly checked while he is in hospital and any R.L.F. will therefore be detected, treated and the parents informed about it.

After leaving hospital there are two **minor** eye troubles that may develop, so an occasional check by an eye specialist is worthwhile. These minor problems are:

Myopia (short-sightedness). This can often be found at a year or so of age and the wearing of glasses later on will satisfactorily correct vision.

Squint (strabismus). Here the eyes do not work together and to the parent it is obvious that sometimes both eyes are not looking in the same direction. This happens in term children too. The eye specialist has a great deal to offer in this situation and results are best if he is able to see and treat the child early.

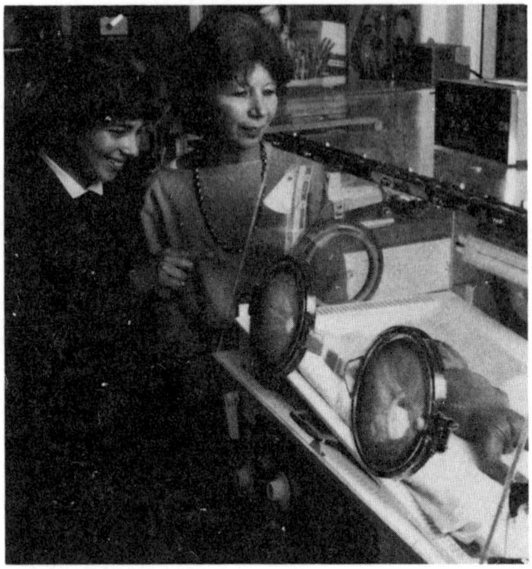

Tanya weighed 940 grams at birth and in this picture she is aged 14 years. She asks her mother "was I really as small as that?"

You may hear a lot of poorly informed talk on eye problems in premature babies. The techniques used in an intensive care unit are designed to reduce eye problems in premature babies to the very minimum. Many years ago it was realized that excessive oxygen was related to eye damage (R.L.F.) in the extremely premature baby. Equally true, insufficient oxygen can result in the loss of a patient, or even survival with some intellectual handicap. The modern use of oxygen greatly reduces the risks of all these conditions.

Intelligence and school performance

Babies less than six weeks premature generally perform quite as well as the family expectation. For the extremely premature baby performance at school is, on average, just a little lower than other members of the family. In practical terms 'just a little' means that a child would be about four places lower down in a class of thirty pupils.

In our experience, a small number of children, while of average intelligence, have memory and perceptual problems which interfere with their learning and recall of symbols such as figures or letters in a word. Now this means that in the classroom situation they have difficulties with math, reading, spelling and sometimes writing. When these problems are not understood children may be unjustly labelled as lazy or inattentive.

Some other children of normal hearing have difficulty discriminating sound against a background noise; thus in the usual busy classroom these children have difficulty in hearing the teacher and so became inattentive in frustration. It is important that teachers and parents understand these problems if they occur so that help, if needed, can be provided early.

Regular visits to your paediatrician or clinic will confirm that all is going well, as is usually the case. If development or school progress is slow, a thorough assessment of the child's pattern of abilities can be made by a psychologist and, if necessary, remedial action taken.

It must be acknowledged that occasionally a premature baby has a severe handicap. This is usually obvious to parents and doctors within a few months of birth. On the brighter side, most children do very well and many who seem to be making rather disappointing progress in the first year or so improve greatly after the age of three years.

Activity, behaviour and attention span

A number of the children are very active and demanding. This is usually a passing phase and parents became generally much happier about behaviour once their child has been at school a year or two. This activity is usually in the normal range and does not require any special medicines or diet. If you are worried, talk to your doctor.

Minor motor incoordination

Some of the young children may be 'clumsy' and poorly coordinated. This shows in such activities as hopping on one foot or carrying out fine tasks with the hands. Again, this slowly improves and usually ceases to worry the parents and child at five to eight years of age.

When to start kindergarten and school?

Kindergarten or pre-school is a learning experience that most children enjoy and we consider it to be especially important to children who were born prematurely. Be sure to enquire about this early and book a place for your child.

The age of commencement at school needs to be considered. Earlier, we referred to the 'corrected age' of a premature baby and this still applies at early school age. Because of the time of year of their birth some children are eligible to start school four and a half years after their actual birthday, yet their age, counted from the expected date of delivery, may be three months younger. A few such children can cope with this first year of school, but some are clearly not ready to begin formal learning. In such cases, the first year may be frustrating and unsatisfactory for child, teacher and parents; indeed it may be an experience that sets the pattern for his future school years.

Once children start school, usually they are promoted each year even if their performance is only marginal. Our advice, therefore, is to delay entry into the primary school until the child is ready and willing to learn. In general, it is better for an ex-premature child to be one of the eldest in the class, rather than one of the youngest. It is much more difficult for the child to have to repeat a grade later because of a premature start to school.

With this caution observed, there should not be many school difficulties. As already mentioned, some children are more active and restless than average and a little clumsy while others have minor memory and perceptual weaknesses. If parents and teachers are aware of these problems early, serious learning problems can be avoided.

The question may be asked: 'Do you tell the teacher that your child was premature?' There are reasons for and against passing on this information. In our experience, if there are any educational problems at all, teachers generally are more interested and helpful when they know the child was premature. More help may be given and in such event the child benefits greatly. However, many parents regard the prematurity of their child as being no business of the school and, if schooling is quite uneventful, this seems a reasonable approach.

Some prematurely born children are still very small in size when they start school. As explained earlier, this probably was because they were small at birth because of the intrauterine growth retardation. In most cases they are not the smallest in the class. Some of the children cope well with their small physical size, but sometimes they and their parents are easily upset by thoughtless remarks about their stature. Medical treatment to improve growth is usually not at all helpful, but you should certainly talk this matter over with your doctor if you are concerned.

CHAPTER 8 Advice when the chances of survival are low

Throughout this book, the expectation has been for the premature baby to live and to go home about the expected date of delivery. Occasionally this happy outcome does not occur. If your baby is more than thirteen weeks premature or weighs under 900 grams (2 pounds) the risk of losing this child is quite high. Very few babies under 600 grams (1 ¼ pounds) or those born more than fifteen weeks early can be saved, even with the most experienced staff and the very best equipment. They are not sufficiently developed when they are born.

It is therefore important to obtain from the intensive care staff a realistic picture of your baby's chances. This sometimes means asking a direct question.

Often in years gone by, parents were given a very gloomy prediction for survival of all premature babies. This was done in the belief that it was best not to arouse feelings of excitement and hope as parents thus would be spared sorrow and grief if the baby died. Although this sounds kind and sensible, real problems may be caused by this approach. When parents assume their baby is going to die, they may commence to grieve in anticipation of his death. In this process of anticipatory grief the parents gradually release their attachment to the child in preparation for their life without him. If the baby recovers the parents have to make a very difficult psychological adjustment of accepting as a living normal person, a baby that in their minds had once died. With improving care of premature babies, more babies who previously would have had little chance of survival now live and grow up normally.

Now let us consider the alternative approach of accepting all babies, no matter how small, as having at least some chance of living. With this attitude realistic expectations are set. Whether their baby lives or not, the parents are comforted by the knowledge that they have done everything possible for the baby right from the beginning. The stage also is set to accept the baby fully if and when the time arrives for coming home.

Parents are advised to see their baby, no matter how premature, and not hold back their love or to fight against the acceptance of this tiny little human being as a member of the family, even if it is not to be for very long.

Most parents are deeply affected by the loss of a very premature baby and recover very slowly. Although this little infant has not had an opportunity to make an impact in society he is a very real person to his parents and he has already been a part of his mother's existence for some months. A large number of people surprise themselves by the depth of their sorrow. It may also come as a surprise to find just how many months this sense of loss and sadness persists.

If you have been unfortunate enough to lose your premature baby, there are a number of ways to make the next few weeks a little more bearable. It may be upsetting and painful to talk with others at this time but there is sure to be someone, your marital partner, minister, a close friend or relative, the social worker, nurse or doctor who will be willing to listen to you. Merely putting thoughts into words and sharing them with others does help.

In coming to terms with death, the finality of it is important to accept. When an older child or adult dies, the ceremony of the funeral and possibly even seeing the person after death releases great emotion and grief which helps towards appreciation of this finality. Later the place of burial and the placing of a memorial emphasize this finality and help towards acceptance of an established fact.

The death of a newborn baby very often is played down in a mistaken belief that a small baby is a small loss. Parents in this situation know better.

Some parents wish to remain with their dying baby, either sitting beside the incubator or cradling the baby comfortably in their arms. Some prefer to do this in a quiet, private place with other family members or close friends also present. Other families may not wish for such a close involvement. The important thing to remember is that you can tell the medical or nursing staff of your wishes and preferences; they will try hard to meet your special needs. If you do not already have a photograph, you might like to ask the staff to take one for you. Some hospitals include a photograph in the hospital records to be given to the parents later if they feel the need for a picture.

Some parents ask to see the baby again after death. If this is your wish, say so. This need not be an unpleasant experience and it again is sometimes helpful in emphasizing the finality of death.

Your doctor may ask the family's permission for post-mortem examination (autopsy). At first this may seem a very callous request at a time of bereavement, but there are always reasons for such a request. The doctor is not always certain of the exact cause of the death and a further examination is the only way of being completely sure. In the future, you will probably want to know the cause of death. If you become pregnant again, the post-mortem result may be very important. Although most troubles do not strike twice, there are some that can recur, and it is important to know the facts. Permission for autopsy may be very important to the future of your family and should not be refused without careful consideration of the advantages.

If you lose a baby, it is often best to leave the hospital as soon as your obstetrician is satisfied with your medical progress. If you need to remain because you are still unwell, you should make certain that you are accommodated where you are least unhappy. Some mothers prefer to stay in the same ward where they already know staff and other mothers, others wish to be in a ward with no mothers and babies, and some wish for a single room where visiting by husband and close relatives can be private and unrestricted.

At home, many normal people have times when the sorrow returns in almost overwhelming severity. These bouts gradually get less intense and less frequent as the weeks go by. Keeping busy and seeing people should help in the meantime. In the first few weeks at home, new questions may occur to you. Why did all this happen? More details of treatment may be needed. What of the prospects for the next pregnancy or indeed is another pregnancy advisable? What about family planning?

It is usual to see either your obstetrician or paediatrician about six weeks after the loss of the baby to ask all these and any other questions that may be troubling you. This is a time when the results of the autopsy will be available and can be discussed. More and more parents expect 'genetic counselling' which is really an attempt to forecast what will happen in the next pregnancy. Ask your doctor about this service if you are interested.

If you have already lost a close relative or friend, the length of time and the intensity of sorrow during the mourning process will be familiar. If this is your first experience with the death of a loved one, successfully coming to terms with death will leave you with new understanding and compassion.

Other help available

Sometimes health professionals do not give you all the help you need. You may have a strong need to talk to a member of the clergy. Also, some hospitals have a social worker who is particularly well qualified to talk to you about matters that are not medical. The social worker will also know about support groups in your city and how to contact one of them. These organizations are formed by those who have personally experienced the death of a baby and some parents feel that only another who has suffered in this way can fully appreciate their feelings. Some booklets are available and the social worker will help find this material if you wish.

Arrangements to be made

Although it may be very painful for parents, arrangements for burial or cremation must be made. Some parents wish for a memorial or religious service to be performed whilst others do not require this. Nursing or medical staff will be able to answer your questions and tell you of the options available and the likely expenses involved. Most hospitals have a pamphlet that explains the details.

Hospital authorities, in an attempt to spare parents further grief and expense may offer to take the responsibility of making the arrangements regarding the funeral. Some parents welcome this offer, but others decide that they must make their own private arrangements for a memorial service and/or funeral. It is best if both parents can discuss these arrangements, rather than one parent making decisions and taking responsibility in the usually mistaken belief that this spares their partner further unnecessary pain.

Even though a baby lives only a few minutes or hours, the birth still must be registered and you will be given another form concerned with registration of the death. Some weeks later you will receive written confirmation that the death has been officially registered.

CHAPTER 9 Follow-up visits to the paediatrician

For the premature baby, visits to the paediatrician may be needed. Babies who were only slightly premature and were not really ill after birth usually need very few follow-up visits. If the infant was very premature, it is usual for the baby to be examined regularly by a paediatrician or in the hospital clinic. This is a routine matter and does not indicate that there is any special concern for your baby.

Why are follow-up visits recommended? There are many good reasons for these regular visits, not the least of which is the opportunity that it provides for the mother to make a list of questions and get authoritative answers. A written list is a good idea; it enables the parents to cross off the items as they get the answers. This saves time.

At the follow-up visits, the baby's weight and length will be checked to see that growth is going well. Baby's progress with smiling, rolling over, crawling, standing and with talking will also be checked to see that these are proceeding as expected.

In the early days the blood may be checked (haemoglobin) at each visit to make sure there is no anaemia of prematurity. (See Chapter 7) Hearing is usually tested as a routine in the first year of life. Likewise an eye specialist is often asked to check the baby regularly as a matter of routine.

Nearly always, the progress is satisfactory and it is reassuring for parents to be told this. In the instance of the few children where development is slow, some positive help is usually available.

How is development assessed?

Development may be assessed in a number of ways. Sometimes it is sufficient for the paediatrician to ask you about the baby's progress and to examine the baby. Some paediatricians carry out a formal developmental test. The most popular is the Denver Developmental Screening Test, which can be done by the doctor but is often done by the parents at home. In some centres a psychologist is available and more complicated tests of physical and intellectual ability can be carried out.

Circumcision

Parents of premature boys often ask about the necessity for circumcision and how soon the operation can be performed.

There are a number of good reasons why a male infant born at the correct time should not be circumcised as a routine. In many developed countries less than half the boys are now being circumcised and in some countries the operation is performed only for religious reasons. If you are anxious to have your boy circumcised, talk over the reasons for and against the operation with your doctor.

If your baby was very premature or sick, it is ill-advised to circumcise him before he leaves hospital. There are risks of infection, bleeding and a poor technical job because of the smaller size of the penis. It will not be medically appropriate to perform a circumcision until he is older. By then he usually needs to have an anaesthetic and this often means a brief admission to hospital. Small wonder that many parents, initially keen to have their baby circumcised, ultimately decide to leave the foreskin as nature intended.

If you decide to have the baby circumcised, your doctor will arrange for this to be done by a competent surgeon with every care taken to make the operation as safe as possible.

These remarks on the timing of the circumcision apply especially to the baby who is more than about four weeks early. If the boy is healthy and only slightly premature, it may be possible to do the operation a little earlier and avoid an anaesthetic, but you will need to be guided by your doctor for his prime concern is safety, not convenience.

Care of the uncircumcised boy

If you decide not to have the baby circumcised, the following information on the care of the uncircumcised child is given for your guidance. Until your boy is at least eighteen months of age, the foreskin is tightly bound to the end of the penis (glans); it has a protective function while the baby is still in diapers most of the time. Do not attempt to pull back (retract) the foreskin of a baby;

this causes him pain and a little bleeding occurs. As well as being unpleasant for all concerned this forcible pulling back of the foreskin may cause scar tissue to form so that a previously perfectly normal child may later need to be circumcised.

Some time around eighteen months to two years the foreskin naturally separates from the tip of the penis and this is often shown by little lumps of yellow, fatty material appearing near the end of the penis. At this age, especially if the lumps of fatty secretion are seen, you may gently try to pull back the foreskin when he is in the bath. Sooner or later the foreskin pulls back painlessly and from now on occasional washing with soap and water is needed. This is far less trouble than washing ears or cleaning finger nails, and you do not have ears removed to save washing!

Some parents ask for their boy to be circumcised because they have heard of the unpleasant experiences of those who were circumcised as adolescents or adults. In these cases circumcision is usually necessary because the foreskin was forcibly retracted in early life. Occasionally a pre-school boy may have an infection under the foreskin as it still will not retract properly. If so, the doctor may recommend circumcision and this is not very disturbing for the four to six year old boy.

In the final analysis, the decision to circumcise or not to circumcise is often made on either religious grounds or because of fixed parental attitudes. Do not assume that all boys must be circumcised. Today more than half are not, but both mother and father will need to discuss the matter with the doctor before arriving at a final decision.

Intervention programmes

It was mentioned earlier that babies who appear to be developing more slowly than expected may be helped by some form of treatment programme. There are a number of early childhood development programmes available; here help with physical development can be provided by a trained physiotherapist and advice on extra intellectual stimulation may also be given. These facilities are intended for those children who are just a little slow in 'getting going' with development.

If the delay in development is more serious, then your paediatrician may suggest a visit to a larger hospital with special facilities or a children's hospital that can check the development of your baby. Here a number of specialists would be involved in the examination of your child. Hearing and eyesight are thoroughly tested and it is usual for a physiotherapist to test the muscular power and coordination of your son or daughter. A paediatrician with special training in assessing development is part of the team. After thorough evaluation, a programme to help your child to progress as quickly as possible will be offered and arrangements made for further visits if you wish.

CHAPTER 10 Multiple Births

This chapter is intended to give you the information you may find helpful around the time of birth of your premature twins or triplets. In this chapter all we say about twins also applies to triplets.

The likelihood of twins varies from country to country, but as a guide, twins may be expected to occur in about one pregnancy in ninety; triplets occur about once in every eight thousand births and quadruplets and quintuplets are very rare indeed. A family history of twins increases the chance of multiple births as does pregnancy immediately after ceasing the long-term use of the contraceptive pill. In addition, in the last few years we have seen more multiple births due to some treatments of mothers for infertility.

In recent times the availability of ultrasound (sonar) means that most multiple births are detected during pregnancy and are therefore expected, but there will always be a few who are surprised. Multiple births are more likely to be premature simply because of the extra size to which the uterus or womb has to stretch. If you and your doctor know you are having twins, together you will be able to plan some extra rest and arrange for the births to take place in a hospital that has special facilities for premature babies and is equipped to deal with any complications that may arise.

Premature twins may have any of the difficulties mentioned in Chapter 3 and a few special ones as well. Your paediatrician or obstetrician would tell you if any of the following apply to your babies.

(a) Sometimes the babies are of very different weights at birth; the smaller baby often loses weight after birth and may need extra feeding to keep the blood sugar (glucose) level normal and some even require intravenous feeding. The smaller twin often remains a little smaller as a child and adult.

(b) Transfusion of blood between twins. Sometimes one twin will be very pale at birth and the other will be a dark red colour; this is because some of the blood from the pale twin has crossed the placenta to the red-coloured twin. If treatment is needed, this will be explained to you.

Feeding

Many mothers successfully breast feed premature twins. Until the babies are sufficiently mature to suck at the breast, it may be necessary to express. Many mothers find this difficult, but patience usually pays off. When the twins are almost ready for home, some mothers will start to feed both babies at the same time; this tandem method saves time. Other mothers cannot immediately achieve a supply that satisfies two babies, but are able to give each twin alternate feeds from the breast and bottle, gradually building up the supply to enable them to continue breast feeding as long as they wish to do so. If you decide not to breast feed, a satisfactory formula is available. Although triplets can be breast fed, many mothers find bottle feeding more practical.

Weight

If the babies are of similar birthweight they are usually ready to go home at the same time. Most parents decide to take both twins home together. This is usually best, but if there are special family circumstances that make this difficult, you should discuss them with the nursery staff.

As mentioned earlier, one baby is sometimes very much smaller and may need to stay in the Special Care Unit for a week or so after the larger baby is ready to go home. Most hospitals are willing and able to keep the twins until both are ready to go home together, but shortage of nurses sometimes makes this impossible. If the smaller twin is not likely to be ready for home for more than ten days, parents often take the bigger one home first. This does enable a first time mother to become accustomed to the routine for one baby and get to know how much help she is going to need when the other twin arrives.

Going home

Parents are often impatient to take their premature twins home just as soon as they possibly can. This is understandable, but because caring for twins is so exacting and tiring for both parents, it is advisable that your babies stay in hospital until they are able to feed vigorously and you and the nursery staff are confident that they are ready to go home.

At home

Most mothers will find it very hard to manage twins without help. The most important, willing and well motivated helper is usually her partner. Parents generally find that this sharing of care of the babies is a very satisfying and rewarding experience. Grandparents and other friends or relatives are sometimes able to help. You should ask about the availability and cost of home-help provided by nurses. These arrangements for assistance should be made before you take the babies home, not when you are desperate for help.

In order that parents have time to enjoy, cuddle and talk to their babies, and not just spend the whole time feeding, washing and changing diapers, it is important to plan time carefully and establish priorities. You may need to restrict yourself to those domestic chores that are absolutely essential. Here a talk with mothers who managed twins will give you the practical suggestions that have worked for them. Twins clubs and or multiple birth associations are to be found in most localities; use the telephone directory or ask at your doctor's office.

Meals for the rest of the family can be simplified and many fathers have hidden catering talents. There are many ways that the work load can be lightened so that you not only look after your babies but also enjoy them.

Visitors

Parents of twins quickly find the babies the centre of attention. Although you will enjoy sharing your pleasure in your children, it is important to be firm with visitors so that they do not arrive unexpectedly or at inconvenient times. You will find that most friends want to be helpful, but may need specific suggestions as to what to do. Do not be diffident about asking for help.

Other children

We mentioned earlier that the other children in the family may become troublesome and behave badly after the birth of a premature baby; this is especially likely to happen if there is not one but two babies. Inevitably parents have less time to spend with older children and the intense interest of visitors in the new babies is usually all too obvious. Parents need to show special love and understanding of their older children to help them through their natural, temporary resentment towards the new babies.

Are our babies identical?

This would seem to be an easy question to answer, but this is not always so. About one third of twins come from a single egg that has divided into two. The resultant twins appear either identical or mirror images of each other. Occasionally they may differ in size, but otherwise they resemble each other so closely that it is very hard to tell them apart. Some parents even need to label their twins at first until they find some little difference, such as a small birthmark, that allows the babies to be identified for certain. While they may look so very much alike it is important to regard them as individuals, each with his own special personality and individual needs.

If two separate fertilized eggs develop, then fraternal twins are produced. Fraternal twins sometimes look obviously different or may be of opposite sexes. However, some fraternal twins resemble each other very closely as is common with brothers and sisters in a family; it is not possible to say whether similar looking twins are either fraternal or identical just by their appearance.

Obstetricians and paediatricians also have difficulty in telling whether twins are identical. Sometimes, but not always, the formation of the after-birth will give them the answer. To be absolutely certain, complicated testing of blood groups of the twins is needed.

What do you tell people who casually ask 'are they identical'? You will probably tire of saying, 'I don't know'. We suggest that if the twins are of the same sex and look very similar you confidently say 'identical'. If they look different or are of opposite sex, say, 'fraternal'. This 'white lie' will save you a lot of pointless explanation.

More advice on the care of twins can be obtained from your obstetrician and paediatrician who will be able to answer many of your questions and will have valuable advice for you.

The National Organization of Mothers of Twins Clubs (5402 Amberwood Lane, Rockville, MD 20853) and La Leche League International have excellent pamphlets; they contain a wealth of practical suggestions for organizing your home so that you not only cope with twins but actually enjoy them. As a new parent of twins, you will think of a lot of these things yourself or learn by experience but advice from these pamphlets and personal advice from parents of twins will often be very helpful.

Conflicting advice

Of one thing you may be quite certain, parents of twins will have no shortage of advice. Very often this advice is conflicting, contradictory or quite impractical. Parents have to make their own decisions with multiple births as they do with single children. For example, it is true that babies can get all the nourishment they require solely from milk until they are at least five months of age; solid foods are **nutritionally** not needed. Yet mothers of hungry sleepless twins in desperation may give some cereal by bottle or spoon at a much earlier age and **sometimes** this works; the babies may sleep a little longer, thus enabling a tired mother to have some rest. Practical solutions may override theoretical considerations.

When one twin wakes up, do you feed them both, even if it means disturbing the other who is sound asleep? We suggest that for some families, it works better to do this, but others and their babies are happier if each is fed when they wake up naturally. **Do you go to bed at night and hope the babies will sleep until midnight or a little later or do you wait up and feed them about 10.00 p.m.?** There is no definite single answer; try the various possibilities and decide which suits you and your babies. Flexibility is the key word.

Breast fed babies can be fed simultaneously; but it may be necessary to have a helping hand at every feed in case one baby loses the nipple and needs help to re-establish sucking.

What about the mother who is bottle feeding? Do you hurry through one bottle feed, leaving the other twin screaming with hunger or do you prop the bottle for one baby and hold the other in your arms? Many will settle for the compromise of propping the bottle; this is less than ideal, but not dangerous if you are in the same room, watching that the baby is feeding comfortably. For many mothers, this is far better than allowing a baby to cry, thus becoming too tired to take the feed when it is finally offered. If it is your decision to prop one baby make sure that equal amounts of nursing and propping are shared between babies.

Parents must decide whether it suits them better for the twins to sleep in another room or at their own bedside. Some professionals will advise against taking the infants into the parents' bed; but again this is a personal decision. Care must always be taken to ensure the baby's safety and comfort.

Being fair

Parents sometimes expect that each twin will need exactly the same amount of affection, attention and cuddling. It is important to realize that every baby is an individual. One twin may demand more attention while the other may be happy with less. It is important to respond to their individual needs, rather than trying to maintain a completely even-handed approach. Try not to make comparisons, two individuals rarely develop in the same way.

The foregoing are just some examples of the early decisions you will have to make. Later on others will arise such as: should you dress the children differently or should you separate them at school? Remember that the methods that suit you and your babies are probably correct for your family. You may need to try the alternatives to decide which you prefer.

Doctors and nurses are able to advise you on the safety, medical and nutritional aspects of child care and you should certainly seek their advice on these matters, but the parents still have to make their own decisions.

CHAPTER 11 The next pregnancy

'What will happen next time?' This is the question often asked after the delivery of a premature baby and the answer will depend very much on the reason for your previous premature delivery. Those who cared for you during your recent pregnancy are best qualified to give you the answer.

A previous premature birth puts you in an 'at risk' group, for it may happen again. The term 'at risk' needs to be looked at more thoroughly; for example, a pedestrian crossing a busy road is 'at risk' of being hit by a passing car. This is not usually a reason for not crossing the road. Precautions such as crossing at traffic lights and looking both ways before crossing to identify the reckless driver make it virtually certain that the road will be safely crossed. For the 'at risk' pregnant woman, extra care greatly increases the prospects for a healthy, mature baby next time.

In this chapter we give some general advice on how to use medical services to your best advantage:

The post-natal visit to the obstetrician

About six weeks after the birth of your baby a check-up by your obstetrician is essential, even if your infant is still in hospital or you have had the misfortune to lose your baby. As part of the check-up your doctor will expect to answer your questions about your future prospects and if or when a further pregnancy is advisable. There will be medical considerations to be talked about. It does help to give your body a rest, especially if you have had two pregnancies in the past two years. Family considerations include the ease or difficulty you may have in becoming pregnant, also your age. Two children both in diapers is an important practical reason for spacing the pregnancies a little.

Any problems with breasts and expressing should be mentioned. If you are not sleeping, still feel depressed or anxious, or if you have any other unusual symptoms, these should be mentioned to your doctor.

If your baby had any abnormality in development, you will probably want to know whether this is likely to occur again. You can sometimes obtain this information either from your

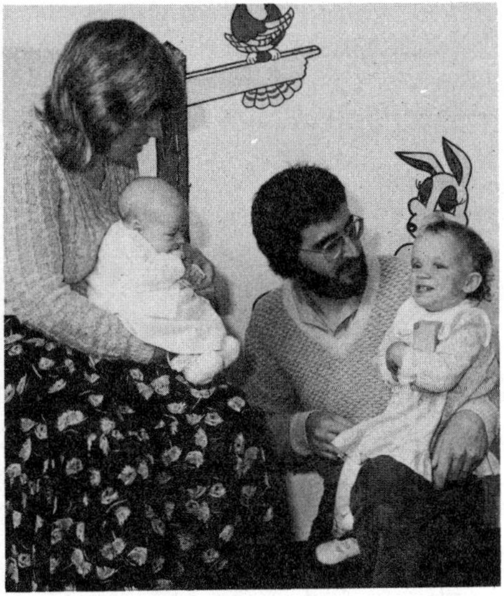

This bright little two year old, Carlie, was 860 grams at birth (less than 2 lbs) (Her first picture is on page 9) Carlie's sister Natalie weighed 3000 g (6 lbs, 10 oz). The family picture was taken when Carlie returned to the hospital for her two year old check-up. She is still small, but bright and talkative.

obstetrician or paediatrician; many parents feel happier if they are referred for genetic counselling from an expert in this field.

Family planning

If you have not already done so then be sure to ask for advice on family planning and contraception at this post-natal visit. Breast feeding or expressing milk certainly does not guarantee that you will not become pregnant.

Choosing your obstetrician and hospital

As the mother of a previous premature baby, it is very important that you receive top quality medical care next time. If possible it would be wise to go to a perinatologist, an obstetrician who specializes in premature and high-risk pregnancies, and arrange for a neonatologist, a paediatrician who handles premature and high-risk newborns, in a hospital with suitable facilities. These hospitals can give you special care during your pregnancy, and should your next baby need special care, this would be available immediately. By taking such precautions, you are doing as much as possible to prevent a possible premature delivery, but also making sure that skilled help for your baby is there if you need it.

We recognize that having your baby in a large, well equipped hospital may be inconvenient because extra travel is required; also, you may prefer the atmosphere of a smaller hospital. As you have already had the experience of a sick or premature baby you will probably decide that your baby's safety is more important than these considerations.

Visit the doctor before starting your next pregnancy

It is important for you to see an obstetrician before you become pregnant again. This visit is especially important if it is the first time you have seen him and he will need to obtain full details of what happened during your previous pregnancy. Attention to general health, weight problems and diet may be needed. The cause of your previous premature delivery, if known, may give a clue to some health problem that requires attention.

Examination of your cervix (neck of womb) when you are not pregnant may suggest that a cervical suture (stitch in the neck of the womb) will be needed quite early in the next pregnancy (see following segment). If so, he will give you more details.

Sometimes other tests are needed before you become pregnant again. If there is an abnormality of the uterus, usually it can be corrected; sometimes other specialists will need to see you too.

It is very important to know when your baby is due, so write down and keep the date of the first day of each period as soon as you decide to become pregnant. Then you will be able to give this vital piece of information, confident that it is accurate.

Care during pregnancy

It is important to see your specialist again as soon as you think you may be pregnant so that pregnancy can be confirmed, a bed booked in the appropriate hospital and plans made for very special care for this important baby.

It is necessary to see your obstetrician early because he may need to check your dates with a 'sonar examination' and this test is most accurate if performed between four and eight weeks of pregnancy. This is painless. It works by bouncing sound waves off the developing baby, which can be seen from a very early stage.

You will be given advice on diet. Cigarette smoking and alcohol are better avoided during pregnancy, but you should ask about these too. Most couples continue with sexual intercourse during pregnancy, but as you had a premature baby last time, you should get the obstetrician's advice on the matter.

Your obstetrician will probably want to see you more often than in a normal pregnancy. At these visits, your cervix (neck of the womb) will be examined regularly to see if a cervical suture is necessary. A cervical suture is not a guarantee that a pregnancy will go to the full time, but for some it certainly helps. The most common time for putting in a suture is between twelfth and sixteenth weeks. Sometimes medications may be needed to stop the uterus from contracting; sometimes even complete rest in bed may be suggested, either in hospital or at home.

Once you have reached 25 weeks of pregnancy, your baby does have a chance of survival and each additional week you gain after that steadily improves the prospects if you come into labour. Normally, your baby is much safer growing in your uterus rather than in an incubator, so if the pregnancy is going well your obstetrician will want to prevent you from delivering until near the due date. If there are reasons for deliberately delivering your baby early, then these will be explained to you.

What to do if you start in labour

If at any time during the pregnancy you begin to feel unusual contractions of the uterus or start to have pains at all like those of labour, don't delay in contacting your obstetrician or else go to the hospital immediately. Any number of false alarms are acceptable if you have a history of premature labour. There is a better chance of stopping labour the earlier the treatment is started. There are drugs that can help to stop the uterus contracting and so put off premature delivery. **Salbutamol** is most commonly used at present; it can be given either by tablet or by intravenous drip. These drugs are not effective in all cases, but often it is possible to keep the pregnancy going for at least a few days and sometimes for many weeks. Again, we would stress that treatment is more likely to succeed if you come to hospital very early in labour.

What to do if the 'waters break' or there is bleeding

If you have any loss of water or blood, even if it is only slight, you should inform your obstetrician or go to the hospital. If the membranes have definitely ruptured (waters break), it is essential that you remain in hospital until the baby is born.

Other general advice

Your obstetrician will give you any special instructions that you need. There are some other things you can do to help the pregnancy to go well. If you are working (outside the home), see if you can cut down the hours or better still, give up work as soon as possible. If not, try to take a leisurely lunch hour, put your feet up, even for a short time and get to bed as early as you can every night.

If you have a small child at home try to take your rest at the same time as the toddler. Make sure you lift the toddler correctly (ask a physiotherapist or midwife to show you how).

When in bed or resting many obstetricians advise mothers to spend as much time as possible lying on their side; in this position more blood circulates through the placenta (after-birth) to give the unborn baby more nourishment, helping him to grow better.

By now you will realize that there are many things you can do to make the next pregnancy a success. Although there are no guarantees, by taking extra precautions yourself and following all instructions given by your obstetrician, you are giving your baby the best possible chance of being born at full time.

Explanation of technical terms

One of the most frustrating and disturbing problems parents may encounter is that of understanding the technical terms used in relation to their premature infant. The parents must suddenly learn a new language that includes concepts and words which may be as foreign to them as a Japanese poem. This may happen at a time of anxiety and worry, a bad time to learn new skills. Ideally this should not be so. It should be possible for health care personnel to make explanations about the baby's condition and his treatment in simple, everyday language. However, in reality this does not always occur and parents may be confused and frightened by communication that is incomprehensible to them. Sometimes this has the effect of closing down communication channels so that parents become diffident about asking more questions and staff are likely to assume their silence indicates understanding. This is an unfortunate situation. Apart from the major consideration of the parents' right to be informed, knowing about the baby's condition, his prospects, keeping up with his treatment are all important ways in which parents relate more closely to their babies and learn to know them.

While efforts are made to have hospital staff communicate clearly with parents without the use of jargon, this is not always achieved: therefore it is useful to become familiar with the terms used in the special care nursery. In any case, in this increasingly technical age many of these words are rapidly becoming part of our everyday language, so some terms will be already familiar and others will be in the future.

To help parents to become familiar with this language of the special care nursery, we are presenting a list of commonly used terms with clarifying explanations. However, if you find yourself confronted with explanations that have no meaning for you or technical words you do not understand, be sure to ask for further clarification. After all, the professionals are talking about your baby and naturally you need to be well informed about him.

Glossary

Acidosis: Excessive acidity, usually applied to the blood. This is common in infants with breathing difficulties.

Alveoli: The small air-containing spaces in the lungs.

Anaemia: Low level of haemoglobin, the red-coloured material in the blood.

Anoxia: Low level of oxygen.

Apgar Score: A simple system for assessing a baby's condition soon after birth, often performed at one and five minutes after birth. The highest score of 10 is very rare in a premature baby and scores of 4 to 7 are quite common.

Apnoea: Not breathing.

Apnoea Alarm Mattress: Machine to warn the staff that a baby's breathing is too slow or too shallow. It may also sound a false alarm if the baby moves around or is very active.

Bilirubin: The yellow-coloured pigment in the blood which colours the skin and whites of the eyes yellow. A blood test to measure the amount present.

Blood Gases: Measurement of the amount of oxygen and carbon dioxide in the blood.

Blood Transfusion: In a simple blood transfusion a small amount of blood is given slowly into a vein; this is often needed to make up for the blood taken from the baby for various blood tests. (See also **Exchange transfusion**).

Bonding: The emotional attachment that develops between parents and baby.

Bradycardia: Slowing of the heart rate. This often occurs during an attack of apnoea.

Bronchopulmonary Dysplasia: Commonly called **B.P.D.**. Damage to lungs, usually temporary, that very commonly occurs in an infant who needs ventilation.

Catheter: This is any sort of tube, usually made of plastic.

Cat-Scan or **C-T Scan:** A special x-ray examination particularly useful in the examination of the brain.

Cervical Incompetence: A condition in the mother in which the neck of the womb (cervix) opens before pregnancy has progressed to the expected time.

Cervix: The lower part or neck of the womb (uterus) which opens into the vagina.

CO_2: Chemical symbol for carbon dioxide, one of the gases present in blood and in the air we breathe out.

C.P.A.P.: Short for the term **Continuous Positive Airway Pressure**. A low pressure is maintained in the lungs to help the baby with breathing difficulty.

Due Date: The date when the baby is expected to be born.

Endotracheal Tube: A tube which passes through either the nose or mouth into the windpipe (trachea).

Exchange Transfusion: A procedure that replaces most of the baby's blood with that of a blood donor. It may be performed either through the umbilical vein at the navel or through blood vessels of the arms or legs.

Fontanelles: These are 'soft spots' in the baby's head; places where the bones have not yet joined together. These soft spots are normal and babies are not hurt by touching them.

Gavage Feeding: For infants who are unable to suck, a thin plastic tube is passed through the mouth or nose into the stomach, then the feeding is slowly poured in. The tube is often left in the stomach all the time if feedings are very frequent.

Gestation: The number of weeks of pregnancy that have passed at the time the baby is born. Normal gestation is 40 weeks.

Growth Retardation: This refers to a slow rate of growth of the unborn baby. Retardation does **not** mean that the baby is mentally retarded.

Haemoglobin: The pigment that gives blood its red colour and helps the blood to carry oxygen. A measure of the amount present.

Head-Box: A convenient way to give a baby extra oxygen.

Hyaline Membrane Disease (H.M.D.): A common cause of difficulty with breathing in a premature baby.

Hydrocephalus: An excessive amount of a watery fluid, usually in the cavities that are always present in the centre of the brain.

Hypoglycaemia: A low level of sugar (glucose) in the blood. This is shown by testing a drop of blood taken from the baby's heel.

Hypoxia: A low level of oxygen in the blood.

Icterus: Jaundice. A yellow colour of the skin (and white part of the eyes) which develops in most premature babies.

Incubator: A machine in which the baby lies so that the temperature of the body is kept at the correct level.

Intensive Care Unit: The small section of the special care unit used for babies who require very close observation or when special equipment is needed.

Intercostal Catheter: A tube inserted into the chest to drain air from a pneumothorax.

Intra-Arterial: Given into an artery.

Intrauterine Growth Retardation (I.U.G.R.): See **Growth Retardation.**

Intravenous Alimentation: Feeding completely or partly by giving a solution of glucose and other nutrients into a vein.

Intraventricular Haemorrhage: Bleeding into the cavities that are situated in the centre of the brain which are normally filled with a watery fluid. It may be detected by sonar.

Jaundice: See **Icterus.**

Kernicterus: A very **rare** complication of **severe** jaundice. Jaundice is treated to prevent kernicterus.

Lanugo: The very fine hair found on the face and body of a premature infant.

Liquor: The watery fluid surrounding the unborn baby.

Low Birthweight: Any baby who weighs 2500 g (5½ pounds) or less at birth. Some babies are premature, others mature but poorly grown.

Meconium: The green material which is always passed from the baby's bowels in the days after birth. Occasionally the baby may pass meconium before birth to give **meconium stained liquor**.

Meningitis: Infection around the brain, a rare condition.

Necrotizing Enterocolitis: An inflamed bowel.

Neonatologist: A paediatrician specializing in premature and high-risk newborns.

Oxygen: The air we all breathe contains about 21 per cent oxygen. Sick infants often need extra oxygen; sometimes even 100 per cent, or pure oxygen may be needed.

Paralysis: Loss of movement of muscles. Some infants are temporarily paralysed with medications because it makes ventilation easier for them.

Perinatologist: An obstetrician specializing in premature and high-risk pregnancies.

Phototherapy: Treatment frequently used for jaundice using light from fluorescent tubes above the baby's incubator.

Placenta: The 'after-birth'. The spongy organ within the uterus which establishes and maintains communication between the mother and her unborn baby by means of the umbilical cord so that nourishment and oxygen can be provided for the developing fetus.

Pneumothorax: The escape of air from the lung into the chest. This causes the lung to collapse. This commonly occurs in an infant on a ventilator.

Pre-Eclampsia (P.E.T.): A complication of pregnancy related to the kidney; the mother may have high blood pressure and swelling of the feet, hands and face.

Premature: Any infant born before the 37th week of pregnancy.

Pre-Term: See **Premature.**

Prone: Lying face downwards.

Respiratory Distress (R.D.S.): Breathing difficulty from any cause. Common in premature infants.

Retrolental Fibroplasia (R.L.F.) A condition developing in the eyes of some premature babies.

Siblings: Brothers and sisters in the same family.

Small-For-Dates (S.F.D.) A baby who is small at birth because of poor growth in the uterus (womb).

Sonar: Sound waves of a very high frequency are often used to produce pictures of such structures as the brain. The examination is safe, painless and non-invasive.

Stridor: Noisy breathing.

Sugar Intolerance: Some babies cannot absorb all the sugar in a normal feed and the bowel actions become very loose and frequent. May be necessary to make the feed weaker or use a special feed.

Supine: Lying on the back.

Surfactant: A substance that lines the alveoli of the lungs. (See **Alveoli**)

T.C.M. or **Transcutaneous Oxygen Monitor:** A device that is put on the baby's skin to determine the oxygen level in blood. It frequently leaves a red mark which fades in a few hours.

Term or **Full-term:** Born at 40 weeks of pregnancy, or 40 weeks' gestation.

Thrush: A common fungal infection causing white patches in the mouth and sometimes a rash in the diaper area. Usually not at all serious. May cause chronically cracked nipples in the mother.

Top-up Transfusions: Giving a small amount of blood, usually to make up for the blood taken for the many tests that a sick baby may need. (See also **Anaemia**.)

Tube Feeding: See **Gavage.**

Ultra Sound: See **Sonar.**

Umbilicus: The navel.

Ventilator: A machine to assist breathing.

Vernix: The white fatty protective coating of the skin — this is not present in the very premature baby.

Viable: Sufficiently mature to be able to live.

Wet-Lung: Breathing difficulty due to too much water in the lungs. This usually improves quickly and is usually not serious.

Further Reading

Boston Women's Health Collective. **Ourselves and Our Children: A Book By and For Parents.** New York: Random House, 1978.

Brewer, Gail Sforza, and Janice Presser Greene. **Right from the Start.** Emmaus, Pa.: Rodale Press, 1981.

Brewster, Dorothy Patricia. **You Can Breastfeed Your Baby . . . Even in Special Situations.** Emmaus, Pa.: Rodale Press, 1979.

Golinsky, Ellen. **Beginnings: A Young Mother's Personal Account of Two Premature Births.** Boston: Houghton Mifflin, 1976.

Haessler, Herbert A. **How to Make Sure Your Baby Is Well . . . and Stays That Way.** New York: Rawson Associates, 1984.

Jones, Sandy. **To Love a Baby.** Franklin Park, Ill.: La Leche League International, 1983.

Kiester, Edwin, Jr., and Sally Valente Kiester. **Better Homes and Gardens New Baby Book.** New York: Bantam, 1982.

La Leche League International. **The Womanly Art of Breastfeeding.** New York: New American Library, 1981; or Franklin Park, Ill.: La Leche League International.

Leach, Penelope. **Baby and Child.** New York: Penguin, 1976.

Leigh, Gillian. **All about Twins.** Boston: Routledge, Kegan, Paul, 1983.

Newton, Niles. **Maternal Emotions.** Franklin Park, Ill.: La Leche League International, 1983.